MRCP PACES
THE ANSWERS REVEALED

Dr Deepa Iyer
MB BS, MRCP(UK), FAFRM(RACP)

Senior Lecturer, Griffith University
Honorary Adjunct Assistant Professor, Bond University

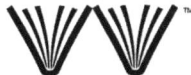

Whiteley Publishing

Published by Whiteley Publishing Ltd
First paperback edition 2022
ISBN 978-1-908586-50-6

The information in this book has been supplied by
the author and has been published by the publisher in
good faith.

Dedicated to my parents,

Dr K Mohan Iyer
My biggest inspiration
and
Mrs Nalini K Mohan
My biggest moral support

Dr Kanishka Banerjee
My loving and caring husband

Vihaan and Kiaan
Our most beautiful sons

Mr Rohit Iyer
My ever-supportive brother

And to all my teachers who believed in me and taught me
the value of perseverance and integrity

Contents

Foreword

Passing PACES is a crucial element in achieving the MRCP(UK) qualification. This is an important milestone for doctors in medical training in the United Kingdom and a very prestigious achievement for many other doctors internationally. This book is an excellent resource for all those preparing for the PACES examination.

The exam assesses 7 clinical skills, including physical examination, Identifying physical signs, communication skills, differential diagnosis, clinical Judgement, managing patient concerns and maintaining patient welfare. These skills that candidates must develop through practice in their day-to-day work are not skills acquired through reading alone. However, to demonstrate these skills, candidates must have the knowledge required depending on the scenario they are being assessed upon. It is here that the book is a very valuable resource for those preparing for the exam.

The author takes the reader through the PACES stations that require clinical examination and identifies most cases that are likely to come up classified under various system headings. The style is clear, straightforward and practical. For each case the author presents, the information that the candidate will most likely need to demonstrate in the exam is noted in point form, under the headings of aetiology, investigation and treatment.

As to direct advice on the informative aspects of the stations, there are often appropriate and important recommendations to the candidates on how to approach the station and other elements to look out for. This makes the book comprehensive yet concise and ideal for studying and revising. This style adopted will keep the book relevant in the future, even if the format of the exam changes. In addition, although the book is intended for PACES candidates, it is also helpful to all candidates preparing for other clinical examinations in Internal Medicine or those simply wanting to refresh their knowledge.

It is a pleasure to provide a foreword for the book by Dr Deepa Iyer, who has already written previous texts on preparing for PACES. In this book, the author's enthusiasm and insight into the subject are evident, and this is a book that I would recommend to all those preparing to sit this exam.

Michael Vassallo
MD, FRCP (Lond) FRCP(Edin) M.Phil, PhD, DGM, F AcadMEd

Consultant Physician and Visiting Professor Bournemouth University

University Hospitals Dorset

July 2022

Preface

It is with great pleasure I wish to present my second book as a follow-up to my first book - 'Clinical examination skills for the MRCP PACES Exam'.

The MRCP exam has become an essential qualifying exam to enter Specialty Training in the NHS. It is crucial for candidates to be aware and thorough with the clinical examination techniques and to be well read on all the common presentations. This helps prove that candidates can take on the responsibilities of a medical registrar.

This book mainly imparts theoretical knowledge to candidates giving this exam. It covers all the common cases and some of the uncommon ones. It provides vital information for every clinical station's most important 4 minutes.

As mentioned in my first book, it is imperative for candidates to practice regularly. Therefore, it is advisable to join a PACES study group and see patients regularly and practice the art of presenting and answering questions.

I hope this humble venture finds favour with all reading it. I wish you all the success in the exam.

Dr Deepa Iyer MB BS, MRCP(UK), FAFRM(RACP)
Senior Lecturer, Griffith University
Honorary Adjunct Assistant Professor, Bond University

Acknowledgements

I would like to extend my most sincere thanks to my family - my parents, husband and brother, who have been the epitome of patience and tolerance while I prepared for this exam.

I would like to thank my consultants and registrars, who spent long hours seeing patients with me and ensuring excellence in my practice.

Finally, I would like to express my most sincere gratitude to all those lovely patients who were so tolerant and compliant and helped me improve my knowledge and skills.

Abdominal System

Case No 1. Chronic Liver Disease

Aetiology

Common Causes

1. Alcoholic liver disease
2. Infections such as hepatitis B and C viruses
3. Autoimmune diseases like primary biliary cirrhosis/ primary sclerosing cholangitis/ autoimmune hepatitis

Other Causes

1. Non-alcoholic steatohepatitis
2. Genetic disorders like alpha-1 antitrypsin deficiency/ hereditary haemochromatosis/ Wilson's disease
3. Drug-induced: e.g. Methyl dopa/ Methotrexate/ Isoniazid/ Phenytoin/ Amiodarone

Management

Investigations

Blood Tests

1. Full blood count
2. Liver function tests and glucose
3. Clotting screen

4. Hepatitis serology
5. Ferritin/ Iron studies
6. Autoantibodies - Anti-nuclear antibodies/ anti-mitochondrial antibodies/ anti-smooth muscle antibodies
7. Alpha-1 antitrypsin
8. Serum ceruloplasmin
9. Alpha-fetoprotein

Imaging Studies

1. Abdominal ultrasound: To look at liver size, texture and vasculature. Also, to assess for ascites
2. MRI Liver: To look more specifically for any lesions/ nodules

Invasive Procedures

1. Ascitic tap if indicated
2. Liver biopsy if indicated

Treatment

General Measures

1. Patient education and advice
2. Encourage good nutrition with a low salt diet
3. Alcohol abstinence
4. Immunisations

Specific Measures

1. If decompensated - consider ascetic tap +/- drain if symptomatic

2. Medications: Treat the cause

    a. Alcohol abstinence - Chlordiazepoxide and Baclofen

    b. Interferon +/- Ribavirin for hepatitis C induced liver disease

    c. Penicillamine for Wilson's disease

    d. Regular venesection and strict iron and haematocrit monitoring for patients with hereditary haemochromatosis

    e. If ascites present - consider spironolactone +/- Furosemide

    f. Consider antibiotics if evidence of spontaneous bacterial peritonitis

3. Always monitor for renal failure - hepatorenal syndrome

4. Ensure multi-disciplinary approach - dietician/ nutritionist/ counsellors/ social worker/ psychologist

5. Liver transplantation

Smart points to remember

1. Child-Pugh Grading of Cirrhosis:

Criteria	Points assigned		
	1	2	3
Ascites	Absent	Slight	Moderate
Bilirubin, mg/dL	</=2	2-3	>3
Albumin, g/dL	>3.5	2.8-3.5	<2.8
Prothrombin time • Seconds over control • INR	1-3 <1.8	4.6 1.8-2.3	>6 >2.3
Encephalopathy	None	Grade 1-2	Grade 3-4

Interpretation

Class	Points	One-year patient survival (%)	Two-year patient survival (%)
A: Well-compensated disease	5-6	100	85
B: Significant functional compromise	7-9	80	60
C: Decompensated disease	10-15	45	35

2. Model for End-stage Liver Disease (MELD):
    - Used for assessing the severity of chronic liver disease

Formula

MELD = 3.78[Ln serum bilirubin (mg/dL)] + 11.2[Ln INR] + 9.57[Ln serum creatinine (mg/dL)] + 6.43

Interpretation

Three months mortality depending on the score:

-   40 or more — 71.3% mortality
-   30–39 — 52.6% mortality
-   20–29 — 19.6% mortality
-   10–19 — 6.0% mortality
-   <9 — 1.9% mortality

Case No 2: Hepatomegaly

Aetiology

Common Causes

1. Mitotic cause - myeloma, leukaemia, lymphoma, secondaries, etc
2. Hepatic congestion secondary to congestive cardiac failure
3. Initial stages of liver cirrhosis

Other Causes

1. Infectious: Infectious mononucleosis, malaria, hepatitis, liver abscess, hydatid cyst
2. Anatomical: Riedels lobe
3. Metabolic causes: Fatty liver, amyloidosis, Gaucher's disease, Nieman Pick disease

Management

Investigations

Blood Tests

1. Full blood count
2. Liver function tests and glucose
3. Clotting screen
4. Hepatitis serology

5. If indicated - thick and thin films
6. Autoantibodies - antinuclear antibodies (ANA), antimitochondrial antibodies (AMA), antineutrophil cytoplasmic antibodies (ANCA), anti-smooth muscle antibodies (ASMA)
7. Immunoglobulins
8. Alpha-fetoprotein
9. Blood cultures

Imaging Studies

1. Chest X-ray – for cardiomegaly
2. ECG
3. Echocardiogram - to assess cardiac function
4. Abdominal ultrasound - to confirm hepatomegaly and to assess the liver size, vasculature and echotexture
5. CT – Chest/ Abdomen and Pelvis - if there is a suspected mitotic lesion
6. MRI Liver

Treatment

General Measures

1. Patient education and advice
2. Encourage good nutrition and exercise
3. Alcohol abstinence
4. Immunisations

Specific Measures

1. Treatment will depend on the cause
2. Mention appropriate referrals to different teams,

ensuring a multi-disciplinary patient management approach.

3. Prompt referral to the oncology team when there is a suspected mitotic lesion to assess for primary or secondary causes.

4. Antibiotics or antiviral therapy as indicated

5. Referral to a cardiologist for prompt management of heart failure

Case No 3: Splenomegaly

Aetiology

Common Causes

1. Chronic myeloid leukaemia (CML)
2. Kala Azar
3. Malaria
4. Myelofibrosis

Other Causes

1. Gaucher's disease
2. Infectious causes - Epstein-Barr virus (EBV), tuberculosis, schistosomiasis
3. Portal hypertension
4. Haematological conditions - CML, lymphoma, haemolytic anaemia
5. Connective tissue disorders - rheumatoid arthritis, systemic lupus erythematosus

Always look out for associated features - arthritis/ weight loss/ generalised lymphadenopathy/ anaemia - will lead you to a differential diagnosis

Management

Investigations

Blood Tests

1. Full blood count and blood film
2. Liver function tests
3. Clotting screen
4. If indicated – thick and thin films
5. Blood cultures

Imaging Studies

1. Chest X-ray - for cardiomegaly
2. ECG
3. Echocardiogram - to assess cardiac function and to look for evidence of vegetations
4. Abdominal ultrasound - to confirm splenomegaly and to assess spleen size, vasculature and echotexture
5. CT - chest, abdomen and pelvis - if a suspected mitotic lesion

Invasive Procedures

1. Bone marrow trephine and biopsy
2. Lymph node biopsy

Treatment

General Measures

1. Patient education and advice
2. Encourage good nutrition and exercise
3. Immunisations

Specific Measures

1. Treatment of any underlying cause
2. If infective - prompt treatment
3. Splenectomy - for hypersplenism, idiopathic thrombocytopenic purpura (ITP), etc
4. Post splenectomy care:

    a. Immunisations - pneumococcal, H influenza type b, meningococcal C and annual influenza vaccine

    b. Lifelong antibiotics - Phenoxymethylpenicillin/ Erythromycin

    c. Medic alert bracelets and splenectomy cards

    d. Prophylactic advice if visiting areas of risk of malaria

    e. Advice to seek medical attention if any signs of infection/ urgent hospital admission in cases of infection for treatment with higher spectrum antibiotics

Case No 4: Hepatosplenomegaly

Aetiology

Common Causes

1. Infective causes - infectious mononucleosis, malaria, leishmaniasis, cytomegalovirus (CMV)
2. Haematological causes: Myeloproliferative disorders, leukaemia, lymphoma, myelofibrosis
3. Chronic liver disease and portal hypertension

Other Causes

1. Amyloidosis
2. Sarcoidosis
3. Systemic lupus erythematosus
4. Acromegaly
5. Gaucher's disease
6. Niemann Pick disease

Management

Investigations

Blood Tests

1. Full blood count and blood film
2. Liver function tests and glucose
3. Clotting screen

4. Hepatitis serology
5. If indicated - thick and thin films
6. Auto antibodies - ANA, AMA, ANCA, ASMA
7. Immunoglobulins and rheumatoid factor
8. Blood cultures

Imaging Studies

1. Chest X-ray - for cardiomegaly
2. ECG
3. Echocardiogram - to assess cardiac function and to look for evidence of vegetations
4. Abdominal ultrasound - to confirm hepatosplenomegaly and to assess liver and spleen size, vasculature and echotexture
5. CT - chest, abdomen and pelvis - if suspected mitotic lesion

Invasive Procedures

1. Bone marrow trephine and biopsy
2. Lymph node biopsy

Treatment

General Measures

1. Patient education and advice
2. Encourage good nutrition and exercise
3. Immunisations

Specific Measures

1. Treatment of any underlying cause

Case No: 5 – Polycystic Kidney Disease

Aetiology

Two types based on genetic prevalence

1. Autosomal Dominant Polycystic Kidney Disease (ADPKD):

    - ADPKD 1 - Chromosome 16

    - ADPKD 2 - Chromosome 4

2. Autosomal Recessive Polycystic Kidney Disease (ARPKD)

It is a progressive, multisystem disorder characterised by the formation of cysts in the kidneys and other organs - spleen, pancreas and liver.

Management

Investigations

Blood Tests

1. Full blood count, hematocrit and blood film
2. Liver function tests
3. Glomerular filtration rate - to stage chronic kidney disease and for monitoring
4. Bone profile - calcium and phosphorus
5. Parathyroid hormone assay
6. Clotting screen

7. Blood cultures - if a suspected infection
8. Genetic testing

Urine Tests

1. Urinalysis
2. Urine culture

Imaging Studies

1. Ultrasound abdomen - to confirm the diagnosis
    a. Remember that if there is a family history present, start screening after the age of 20 years unless symptomatic
2. CT, MRI and MRA may be useful in certain cases

Treatment

General Measures

1. Patient education and advice
2. Encourage good nutrition and exercise
3. Immunisations

Specific Measures

1. Treat hypertension promptly
2. Monitor for renal failure and treat urine infections and hematuria promptly
3. Regular neurological examination if a history of subarachnoid bleeds
4. Consider renal replacement therapy - hemodialysis/ peritoneal dialysis/ renal transplantation
5. Monitor for metabolic problems and treat promptly

Case No 6: Organ Transplants – Liver/ Kidney/ Pancreas/ Other

Indications for Liver Transplant

Acute Indications

1. Fulminant acute hepatic necrosis secondary to:
   - Drug toxicity like salicylate poisoning
   - Viral hepatitis
   - Toxins

Chronic Indications

1. Chronic liver disease secondary to:
   - Alcoholic liver disease
   - Cholestatic diseases like primary biliary cirrhosis, primary sclerosing cholangitis
   - Chronic hepatitis secondary to hepatitis B, hepatitis C, hepatitis D, chronic active Hepatitis
   - Metabolic diseases like haemochromatosis, Wilson's disease, alpha-1 antitrypsin deficiency, glycogen storage disorders
   - Sometimes, for primary liver tumours like hepatocellular carcinoma

Indications for a Kidney Transplant

Causes for end-stage renal disease (GFR<15ml/min):

- Diabetes
- Hypertension
- Polycystic kidney disease
- Glomerulonephritis

Indication for Simultaneous Pancreas - Kidney Transplant (SPK)

Type 1 diabetes with renal failure from diabetic nephropathy

Types of organ transplants

1. Allograft: Transplant of organ or tissue from genetically non-identical members of the same species.
2. Autograft: Transplants of tissue to the same person.
3. Isograft: Transplants of organs or tissue from a genetically identical donor.
4. Xenograft: Transplants of tissue from one species to another

Types of organ donors

1. Living donors
2. Deceased or cadaveric donors

Teams involved in organ transplantation

1. Transplant medical specialist
2. Transplant surgeon

3. Transplant nurse co-ordinator
4. Transplant psychological services
5. Transplant pharmacists
6. Clinical dieticians
7. Transplant financial counsellors
8. Procurement co-ordinators

Post transplantation care

1. Medications - mainly immunosuppressants:
   - Induction immunosuppression
   - Maintenance immunosuppression
   - Anti-rejection immunosuppression

2. Promoting a healthy lifestyle post-transplant:
   - Post-transplant follow-up with regular tests
   - Monitor and prevention of rejection
   - Ensure a healthy diet with adequate exercise
   - Monitoring for infections and prompt treatment

3. Ensure that patients have been given details and contacts for further advice, including emergency numbers and support services

4. Multi-disciplinary approach to ensure a return to work and lifestyle modifications

5. Prompt monitoring for cancer associated with transplants

6. Prompt monitoring of drug levels and ensuring a check on side effects and toxicities

Case No 7: Haemochromatosis

Aetiology

It is a genetic disorder causing the body to absorb excessive iron from the diet. This absorbed iron is then deposited in various organs, mainly in the liver but other organs targeted are the pancreas, joints, heart and endocrine glands.

Inheritance
- Type 1, 2 and 3 haemochromatoses: Inherited as autosomal recessive
- Type 4: Autosomal dominant

Genetic Mutations

Mutations in HAMP, HFE, HFE2, SLC40A1 and TFR2 genes cause haemochromatosis.

Management

Investigations

Blood Tests

1. Full blood count
2. Liver function tests
3. Iron studies
4. Transferrin saturation
5. Serum ferritin

6. Blood glucose and HbA1C
7. Genetic test looking for the HFE gene mutation

Imaging Studies

1. X-rays of painful joints
2. Echocardiography

Invasive Procedures

1. Liver biopsy

Treatment

General Measures

1. Patient education and advice
2. Ensure healthy eating habits and exercise
3. Monitor for diabetes and prompt referral to the diabetic services
4. Annual vaccinations

Specific Measures

1. Venesection or phlebotomy - initially once or twice weekly, then once a month, once ferritin levels are acceptable - 20 micrograms/l
2. Once ferritin levels are under control - venesection may be required 3 - 4 monthly.
3. Low iron diet
4. Avoid alcohol
5. Avoid vitamin supplements/ diet/ medications containing iron.
6. Iron chelators are sometimes used

7. Liver transplantation in end-stage liver disease
8. Regular monitoring of haemoglobin, haematocrit and serum ferritin is critical

Case No 8: Primary Biliary Cirrhosis

A chronic and progressive cholestatic disease of the liver.

Important Points to Remember

1. Aetiology unknown - presumed auto-immune disease
2. Commonly affects middle-aged women
3. Fatigue, generalised pruritis and right upper quadrant pain are the common presentations
4. Features of chronic liver disease on examination

Management

Investigations

Blood Tests

1. Full blood count
2. Liver function tests and glucose
3. Clotting screen
4. Hepatitis serology
5. Ferritin/ iron studies
6. Autoantibodies - ANA/ AMA/ ASMA
7. Alpha-1 antitrypsin
8. Serum ceruloplasmin
9. Alpha-fetoprotein
10. Immunoglobulins - IgM - M2 subtype

Imaging Studies

1. Abdominal ultrasound: To look at liver size, texture and vasculature. Also, to assess for ascites.
2. MRI Liver: To look more specifically for any lesions/nodules

Invasive Procedures

1. Ascitic tap if indicated
2. Liver biopsy if indicated

Treatment

General Measures

1. Patient education and advice
2. Encourage good nutrition with a low salt diet
3. Alcohol abstinence
4. Immunisations

Specific Measures

1. If decompensated - consider ascetic tap +/- drain if symptomatic
2. Medications:
    a. To alleviate the symptoms hence slowing the progression of the disease - ursodeoxycholic acid
    b. Immunosuppressive therapy, corticosteroids
    c. For pruritis: Cholestyramine, Rifampicin
    d. Plasmapheresis
3. Treat the underlying auto-immune condition
4. Ensure multi-disciplinary approach - dietician/nutritionist/ counsellors/ social worker/ psychologist
5. Liver transplantation

Case No 9: Inflammatory Bowel Disease

Types

1. Ulcerative colitis - limited to the colon
2. Crohn's disease - can involve any part of the gastrointestinal tract from mouth to anus.

Aetiology

1. Unknown
2. Genetic, infectious, immunological and psychological factors are implicated.

Management

Investigations

Blood Tests

1. Full blood count
2. Liver function tests
3. Iron studies
4. Renal function
5. Infection screen
6. If there is a history of heavy bleeding - group and save
7. Stool - microscopy, culture and sensitivities

Imaging Studies

1. Barium swallow and barium enema
2. Upper gastrointestinal (GI) endoscopy and colonoscopy

Invasive Procedures

1. Colonic biopsy

Treatment

General Measures

1. Patient education and advice
2. Encourage good nutrition and exercise
3. Immunisations

Specific Measures

1. First-line agents include aminosalicylates - e.g., Sulphasalazine, Olsalazine - these can be administered orally or rectally
2. Corticosteroids - depending on severity - Methylprednisolone, Hydrocortisone, Prednisolone - fast-acting anti-inflammatory drugs.
3. Immunomodulators - 6-Mercaptopurine analogues, Azathioprine
4. Anti-TNF drugs - Infliximab
5. Antibiotics: Metronidazole, Ciprofloxacillin
6. Symptomatic treatments: Drugs against diarrhoea, antispasmodic and antacids

Case No 10: Nephrotic Syndrome

Triad: Proteinuria, hypoalbuminemia, and oedema

Aetiology

1. Primary Renal Causes

    a.   Minimal change nephropathy

    b.   Focal glomerulosclerosis

    c.   Membranous nephropathy

2. Other Causes

    a.   Diabetes

    b.   Viral infections - e.g., hepatitis B and C, human immunodeficiency virus (HIV)

    c.   Amyloidosis and paraproteinemia

Management

Investigations

Blood Tests

1. Full blood count, hematocrit and blood film
2. Liver function tests
3. Bone profile - calcium and phosphorus
4. Lipid profile
5. Clotting screen

6. Immunoglobulins
7. Fasting blood sugar/ HbA1C
8. Infectious screen - hepatitis serology, HIV
9. Auto immune screen - ANA, ANCA, Anti dsDNA, etc

Urine Tests

1. Urinalysis
2. Urine culture
3. Protein-creatinine ratio

Imaging Studies

1. Ultrasound abdomen

Invasive Procedures

1. Renal biopsy

Treatment

General Measures

1. Patient education and advice
2. Encourage good nutrition and exercise
3. Immunisations
4. Regular diabetic checks

Specific Measures

1. Treatment of any underlying cause
2. Treatment of diabetes
3. Acute management with diuretics, anticoagulation,

lipid-lowering therapy, ACE inhibitors/
angiotensin-2 receptor antagonists

4. Steroids - Prednisolone
5. Calcium and vitamin D supplementation
6. Immunomodulators:
   Cyclophosphamide, Ciclosporin and Rituximab
7. Immunosuppressants: Mycophenolate

Respiratory System

Case No 1: Interstitial Lung Disease

Introduction

Interstitial lung disease is one of the commonest cases in the respiratory station. It refers to a broad category of conditions affecting the pulmonary interstitium.

Aetiology

1. Idiopathic: Cause unknown

2. Rheumatological Conditions
   a. Rheumatoid arthritis
   b. Systemic lupus erythematosus
   c. Polymyositis
   d. Dermatomyositis
   e. Systemic sclerosis

3. Occupational
   a. Berylliosis
   b. Asbestosis
   c. Silicosis
   d. Coal workers pneumoconiosis

4. Iatrogenic/ Drug-induced
   a. Amiodarone

b. Methotrexate

c. Nitrofurantoin

d. Busalphan

e. Statins

5. Others

a. Tuberculosis

b. Sarcoidosis

c. Radiation fibrosis

d. Allergic bronchopulmonary aspergillosis

Management

Investigations

Blood Tests

1. Full blood count

2. Liver function tests

3. Renal function

4. Erythrocyte sedimentation rate (ESR)

5. C-reactive protein (CRP)

6. Rheumatological profile - including a vasculitic screen

7. Aspergillus

8. QuantiFERON gold for tuberculousis (TB)

9. Arterial blood gases

Imaging Studies

1. Chest X-ray - reticular/ nodular opacities

2. High-resolution CT scan of the thorax - could range from normal to ground glass changes to

honey combing in the late stages

Others

1. ECG
2. Echocardiogram - to look for evidence of pulmonary hypertension
3. Spirometry and Lung volumes: Shows a restrictive pattern with a reduced transfer factor

Invasive Procedures

1. Transbronchial or endobronchial biopsy
2. Bronchoalveolar lavage
3. Video-assisted thoracic lung biopsy

Treatment

General Measures

1. Patient education and advice
2. Smoking cessation
3. Annual vaccinations
4. Avoidance of the cause if iatrogenic
5. Healthy diet and exercise
6. Pulmonary rehabilitation

Specific Measures

1. Refer to a respiratory physician
2. Oxygen therapy if hypoxic
3. Corticosteroids
4. Antifibrotic treatment with Colchicine, D Penicillamine, Ciclosporin

5. Steroid sparing agents - Methotrexate, Cyclophosphamide, Azathioprine
6. Lung transplantation

Types: American Thoracic Society and European Respiratory Society (ATS/ERS) Classification

1. UIP (Usual Interstitial Pneumonia), the most common, insidious onset, chronically progressive, usually does not respond to therapy and is fatal in most cases.

2. NSIP (Non-specific Interstitial Pneumonia) does not fit histologically with any other idiopathic interstitial pneumonia. Interstitial inflammation is often prominent, the prognosis is generally good, and it responds to steroids in most patients.

3. COP (Cryptogenic Organising Pneumonia)

4. AIP (Acute Interstitial Pneumonia) (Hamman-Rich Syndrome) is an acute, fulminant, severe, extensive acute lung injury, rapid course, evolving over several months, and has a high mortality rate.

5. DIP (Desquamative Interstitial Pneumonia), rare form, insidious onset, good prognosis. It may be related to cigarette smoking.

6. RB-ILD (Respiratory Bronchiolitis associated Interstitial Lung disease)

7. LIP (Lymphoid Interstitial Pneumonia)

Case No 2: Bronchiectasis

Definition

Bronchiectasis is a chronic suppurative condition affecting the lungs secondary to an infectious process that results in an abnormal and permanent dilatation of one or more of the conducting airways or bronchi.

Aetiology

Congenital Causes

1. Kartagener's syndrome
2. Cystic fibrosis
3. Young's syndrome
4. Alpha-1 antitrypsin deficiency
5. Primary immunodeficiencies

Acquired Causes

1. Childhood infections - measles, pertussis, etc
2. Tuberculosis
3. Aspiration pneumonia
4. Allergic bronchopulmonary aspergillosis
5. Acquired immunodeficiency syndrome

Management

Investigations

Blood Tests

1. Full blood count
2. Liver function tests
3. Renal function
4. ESR
5. CRP
6. Rheumatological profile - including a vasculitic screen
7. Aspergillus
8. QuantiFERON gold for TB
9. HIV test
10. Immunoglobulins
11. Alpha-1 antitrypsin levels
12. Pilocarpine iontophoresis - sweat test
13. Aspergillus precipitins and IgE levels
14. Arterial blood gases

Sputum – for microscopy, culture and sensitivity

Imaging Studies

1. Chest X-ray
2. High-resolution CT scan of the thorax – honeycomb changes, signet ring appearance, tram track lines, etc.

Others

1. ECG
2. Echocardiogram - to look for evidence of pulmonary

hypertension

3. Spirometry and Lung volumes: Shows an obstructive pattern

Invasive Procedures

1. Bronchoscopy

Treatment

General measures

1. Patient education and advice
2. Smoking cessation
3. Annual vaccinations - especially confirming immunisation to mumps, measles and pertussis
4. Avoidance of the cause if iatrogenic
5. Healthy diet and exercise
6. Pulmonary rehabilitation

Specific measures

1. Refer to a respiratory physician
2. Oxygen therapy if hypoxic
3. Antibiotic therapy - consider long-term antibiotics
4. Corticosteroids
5. Bronchodilator therapy
6. Anti-inflammatory therapy - steroids, non-steroid anti-inflammatory agents, leukotriene receptor antagonists
7. Surgical resection
8. Lung transplantation
9. Long-term respiratory follow-up

Case No: 3 – Pleural Effusion

Definition

A pleural effusion is an abnormal collection of fluid in the pleural space, either from increased production or decreased absorption results in a pleural effusion.

Aetiology

Exudative Effusion

1. Infectious causes - parapneumonic effusions
2. Malignancy
3. Pulmonary embolism
4. Trauma
5. Oesophageal perforation
6. Pancreatitis

Transudative Causes

1. Congestive cardiac failure
2. Chronic liver disease
3. Chronic renal failure
4. Nephrotic syndrome
5. Hypoalbuminemia

Management

Investigations

Blood Tests

1. Full blood count
2. Liver function tests
3. Renal function
4. ESR
5. CRP
6. Rheumatological profile - including a vasculitic screen
7. Aspergillus
8. QuantiFERON gold for TB
9. HIV test
10. Immunoglobulins
11. Alpha-1 antitrypsin levels
12. Arterial blood gases

Imaging Studies

1. Chest X-ray - PA and lateral views
2. Ultrasound thorax - to quantify and mark the effusion
3. CT Thorax

Other Investigations

1. Sputum - for microscopy, culture and sensitivity

Invasive Procedures

1. Thoracocentesis - pleural aspiration for diagnostic purposes or a therapeutic drain for symptomatic effusions.

Send Pleural Fluid for

- Biochemistry: Protein, LDH, albumin, ph, amylase and glucose
- Microscopy and culture - including gram stain
- Cell count, differential cell count and cytology
- Others: Lipids, immunoglobulins, etc

Normal pleural fluid has the following characteristics

- A pH of 7.60 - 7.64
- Protein content of less than 2% (1 - 2 g/dL)
- Fewer than 1000 white blood cells per cubic millimetre
- Glucose content similar to that of plasma
- Lactate dehydrogenase less than 50% of plasma

Light's Criteria: To help distinguish between transudative and exudative effusions

1. The ratio of pleural fluid protein to serum protein is greater than 0.5
2. The ratio of pleural fluid LDH and serum LDH is greater than 0.6
3. Pleural fluid LDH is greater than 0.6 or $2/3$ times the normal upper limit for serum.

NB: Different laboratories have different values for the upper limit of serum LDH

2. Bronchoscopy
3. Thoracoscopy
4. Pleural biopsy
5. Open lung biopsy

Treatment

General Measures

1. Patient education and advice
2. Smoking cessation
3. Annual vaccinations - especially confirming immunisation to mumps, measles and pertussis
4. Avoidance of the cause, if iatrogenic
5. Healthy diet and exercise
6. Pulmonary rehabilitation

Specific Measures

1. Refer to a respiratory physician
2. Oxygen therapy if hypoxic
3. Therapeutic drainage if symptomatic
4. Antibiotic therapy
5. Pleurodesis - for recurrent effusions
6. VATS - Video Assisted Thoracoscopic Surgery
7. Treatment of any underlying cause

Case No 4: Pneumonectomy/ Lobectomy/ Lung Transplant

Indications for Pneumonectomy/ Lobectomy

1. Malignancy
2. Tuberculosis
3. Bronchiectasis

Indications for Lung Transplantation

1. End-stage COPD
2. Idiopathic pulmonary fibrosis
3. Pulmonary hypertension
4. Cystic fibrosis
5. Others: Sarcoidosis, bronchiectasis

Management

Investigations

Blood Tests

1. Full blood count
2. Liver function tests
3. Renal function
4. ESR
5. CRP
6. Rheumatological profile - including a vasculitic

screen

7. QuantiFERON gold for TB
8. HIV test
9. Immunoglobulins
10. Alpha-1 antitrypsin levels
11. Arterial blood gases

Treatment

General Measures

1. Patient education and advice
2. Smoking cessation
3. Annual vaccinations - especially confirming immunisation to mumps, measles and pertussis
4. Healthy diet and exercise
5. Pulmonary rehabilitation

Specific Measures

1. Refer to a respiratory physician
2. Monitor for immunosuppressant side effects
3. Long term follow up

Case No 5: Chronic Obstructive Airways Disease

Definitions

1. **Chronic bronchitis** is the presence of a chronic productive cough for at least 2 months in 2 consecutive years, excluding other causes for a chronic cough.

2. **Emphysema** is a pathologically abnormal, permanent enlargement of the airspaces distal to the terminal bronchioles, associated with the destruction of their walls without evidence of obvious fibrosis.

3. **Chronic Obstructive Airways Disease** is a progressive airflow obstruction, not fully reversible and does not change markedly over several months.

Aetiology

1. Smoking
2. Environmental factors: Exposure to traffic-related air pollution, use of biomass fuels with indoor cooking and heating.
3. Alpha-1 antitrypsin deficiency
4. Bronchial hyperreactivity
5. Connective tissue disorders - Marfan's Syndrome, Ehlers-Danlos Syndrome

Management

Investigations

Blood Tests

1. Full blood count
2. Liver function tests
3. Renal function
4. ESR
5. CRP
6. Rheumatological profile - including a vasculitic screen
7. Aspergillus
8. QuantiFERON gold for TB
9. HIV test
10. Immunoglobulins
11. Alpha-1 antitrypsin levels
12. B-Type Natriuretic peptide - to distinguish from heart failure
13. Arterial blood gases

Imaging Studies

1. Chest X-ray
2. CT chest
3. Echocardiogram - to look for pulmonary hypertension

Other Investigations

1. Six-minute walking distance test
2. Sputum - for microscopy, culture and sensitivity
3. ECG

4. Lung Function tests:

- Airflow obstruction is defined as a reduced post-bronchodilator FEV1/FVC ratio, such that FEV1/FVC is less than 0.7 (FEV1 – Forced Expiratory Volume in 1 second, FVC – Forced Vital Capacity)

- If FEV1 is more than or equal to 80% predicted normal, a diagnosis of COPD must be made only in the presence of respiratory symptoms like breathlessness or cough.

Severity grading according to NICE clinical guideline - 2010

Post-bronchodilator FEV1/FVC	FEV1 % predicted	Post bronchodilator severity
< 0.7	>/= 80%	Stage 1 - Mild
< 0.7	50 - 79%	Stage 2 - Moderate
< 0.7	30 - 49%	Stage 3 - Severe
< 0.7	<30%	Stage 4 - Very severe

Treatment

General Measures

1. Patient education and advice
2. STOP SMOKING!!
3. Encourage physical activity/ exercise
4. Annual influenza vaccination and offer pneumococcal vaccination
5. Dietician review for nutritional support

6. Psychologist review for anxiety and depression
7. Physiotherapy and occupational therapy services
8. Social services

Specific Measures

1. Refer to a respiratory physician
2. Start with short-acting beta-agonists (SABA) or short-acting muscarinic antagonists (SAMA)
3. If patients continue with exacerbations or persistent breathlessness:
   - If FEV1 >/= 50%
   - Add a long-acting beta-agonist (LABA)
   - Add a long-acting muscarinic antagonist (LAMA) and stop the SAMA
   - If FEV1 <50%
   - Add a LABA with inhaled corticosteroids (ICS) in a combination inhaler
   - Consider LABA + LAMA if ICS declined or is not tolerated
   - Add LAMA and discontinue SAMA
4. If patients continue to have persistent exacerbations or breathlessness:
   - Try the LABA with ICS in a combination inhaler
   - Add LAMA with LABA+ICS in a combination inhaler
5. Patients may need hospitalisation for acute exacerbations
6. Antibiotics and steroids along with nebulisation for infective exacerbations
7. Non-Invasive ventilation: For persistent

hypercapnic respiratory failure during exacerbations after optimal medical therapy.

8. Long-term oxygen therapy (LTOT):

   Assess the need for LTOT in patients with:

   - Very severe airflow obstruction (FEV1<30% predicted)
   - Cyanosis
   - Polycythaemia
   - Peripheral oedema
   - A raised Jugular venous pressure
   - Oxygen saturation less than or equal to 92% breathing air

Offer LTOT to patients with PaO2 less than 7.3kPa when stable, or greater than 7.3 and less than 8kPa when stable and:

   - Secondary polycythaemia
     OR
   - Nocturnal hypoxaemia
     OR
   - Peripheral oedema
     OR
   - Pulmonary Hypertension

8. Consider other causes of COPD and treat accordingly

9. Consider mucolytic therapy for chronic productive cough

10. Osteoporosis prophylaxis for patients on long-term steroids

11. All patients should be enrolled in pulmonary

rehabilitation

12. Surgery: Lung volume reduction surgery/ bullectomy/ lung transplantation

13. Regular specialist follow-up and referral to multi-disciplinary palliative care teams and hospices when appropriate.

Case No 6: Mitotic Lung Lesion

Introduction

Classification

1. Non-small cell lung cancer:
    a. Adenocarcinoma
    b. Squamous cell cancer
    c. Large cell cancer

    Staging using TNM staging (from American Joint Committee on Cancer (AJCC))

2. Small cell lung cancer

    Staging as - Limited and extensive

Management

Investigations

Blood Tests

1. Full blood count
2. Liver function tests
3. Renal function
4. ESR
5. CRP
6. Rheumatological profile - including a vasculitic screen
7. Aspergillus

8. QuantiFERON gold for TB
9. HIV test
10. Arterial blood gases

Imaging Studies

1. Chest X-ray
2. CT chest along with Abdomen and pelvis - as the initial staging scan
3. Echocardiogram

Others

1. Lung function tests
2. Sputum - for microscopy, culture and sensitivity
3. ECG

Invasive Procedures: For Tissue Diagnosis

1. Bronchoscopy
2. CT guided biopsy

Treatment

General Measures

1. Patient Education and advice
2. STOP SMOKING!!
3. Encourage physical activity/ exercise
4. Annual influenza vaccination and offer pneumococcal vaccination
5. Dietician review for nutritional support
6. Psychologist review for anxiety and depression

7. Physiotherapy and occupational therapy services
8. Social services

Specific Measures

1. Refer to a respiratory physician and oncologist
2. Options for treatment depend on histology
    a. Chemotherapy
    b. Radiotherapy
    c. Chemo and radiotherapy
    d. Surgery
    e. Palliative measures in case of advanced or metastatic disease not amenable to chemo or radiotherapy
3. Involve a multi-disciplinary team from the start
4. Regular specialist follow-up and referral to multi-disciplinary palliative care teams and hospices when appropriate
5. Monitor for treatment-associated side effects

Case No 7: Cystic Fibrosis

Introduction

Cystic fibrosis is an autosomal recessive genetic disorder affecting the exocrine function and involving multiple organs, including the lungs, pancreas, liver and intestine.

Cystic fibrosis is caused by defects in the cystic fibrosis gene, which codes for a protein transmembrane conductance regulator (CFTR) that functions as a chloride channel and is regulated by cyclic adenosine monophosphate (cAMP). Mutations in the CFTR gene result in abnormalities of cAMP-regulated chloride transport across epithelial cells on mucosal surfaces. ΔF508 is the most common mutation detected.

Management

Investigations

Blood Tests

1. Full blood count
2. Liver function tests
3. Renal function
4. ESR
5. CRP
6. Rheumatological profile - including a vasculitic screen

7. Aspergillus
8. QuantiFERON gold for TB
9. HIV test
10. Immunoglobulins
11. Alpha-1 antitrypsin levels
12. Pilocarpine iontophoresis - sweat chloride test
13. Aspergillus precipitins and IgE levels
14. Arterial blood gases
15. Genetic testing
16. Immunoreactive trypsinogen

Imaging Studies

1. Chest X-ray
2. High-resolution CT scan of the thorax

Other Investigations

1. Sputum - for microscopy, culture and sensitivity
2. ECG
3. Echocardiogram - to look for evidence of pulmonary hypertension
4. Spirometry and lung volumes: Shows an obstructive pattern with air trapping and hyperinflation

Invasive Procedures

1. Bronchoscopy - Bronchoalveolar lavage with sputum microbiology

Treatment

General Measures

1. Patient education and advice
2. Smoking cessation
3. Annual vaccinations - especially confirming immunisation to mumps, measles and pertussis
4. Healthy diet and exercise
5. Pulmonary rehabilitation
6. Multi-disciplinary involvement - Physiotherapists, occupational therapists, dieticians, psychologists, and social workers.

Specific Measures

1. Refer to a respiratory physician
2. Oxygen therapy if hypoxic
3. Antibiotic therapy - consider long-term antibiotics
4. Corticosteroids
5. Bronchodilator therapy, mucolytics
6. Anti-inflammatory therapy - steroids, non-steroid anti-inflammatory agents, leukotriene receptor antagonists
7. Chest physiotherapy with postural drainage
8. Pancreatic enzyme supplements, multivitamins
9. Newer agents - CFTR potentiator - Ivacaftor
10. Surgical resection
11. Lung transplantation
12. Long-term respiratory follow-up
13. Specialist follow-up as appropriate - Cardiologist, gastroenterologist, transplant team, etc.

Case No 8: Old Tuberculosis

Introduction

Tuberculosis (TB) is a multisystem disease with many presentations associated with morbidity and mortality.

Causative Organism: Mycobacterium tuberculosis

In the MRCP Exam, we do not expect active cases of tuberculosis. Hence any patients with tuberculosis will have received treatment in the past. However, old tuberculosis could be a differential diagnosis for a patient with evidence of fibrosis. It is also more likely if the patient has scars suggestive of thoracoplasty, plombage, phrenic nerve crush or induced pneumothorax.

Management

Investigations

Blood Tests

1. Full blood count
2. Liver function tests
3. Renal function
4. ESR
5. CRP
6. Rheumatological profile - including a vasculitic screen

7. Aspergillus
8. HIV
9. Blood cultures
10. Arterial blood gases

Screening Tests

1. Mantoux test with purified protein derivative for active or latent infection
2. Interferon-gamma release assay for latent infection
3. Sputum for acid-fast bacilli smear and culture

Imaging Studies

1. Chest X-ray
2. High-resolution CT scan of the thorax

Also, consider work-up for extra pulmonary TB

1. Lumbar puncture - in suspected tuberculous meningitis
2. CT/MRI Spine if suspected Pott's disease of the spine
3. Urine microscopy, culture and sensitivity in cases of genitourinary symptoms
4. Biopsy of liver/ bone marrow, if indicated

Treatment

General Measures

1. Patient education and advice
2. Smoking cessation
3. Annual vaccinations

4. Healthy diet and exercise
5. Pulmonary rehabilitation
6. Multi-disciplinary involvement - Physiotherapists, occupational therapists, dieticians, psychologists, and social workers.

Specific Measures

1. Refer to a respiratory physician
2. Isolation of patient until 3 sputum smears are negative
3. Initial empiric treatment with Isoniazid, Rifampicin, Pyrazinamide and Ethambutol - 2 months of intensive phase
4. Continuation phase with Isoniazid and Rifampicin for 4 – 7 months
5. Monitor for side effects of treatment, drug resistance, compliance, complications
6. Surgical resection may be considered in some cases.
7. Long-term monitoring for complications, including relapse

Case No 9: Rheumatoid Lung

Introduction

Rheumatoid arthritis is a multisystem disorder needing specialist involvement from very early stages to prevent extra-articular manifestations.

Rheumatoid arthritis could cause any of the problems mentioned above. From pleural disease to fibrotic lung disease, the presentation is diverse.

The major varieties of pulmonary manifestations include:

1. Pleural effusion
2. Nodular lung disease
3. Diffuse interstitial fibrosis
4. Pulmonary vasculitis
5. Alveolar haemorrhage
6. Obstructive pulmonary disease
7. Infections

Management

Investigations

Blood Tests

1. Full blood count
2. Liver function tests
3. Renal function
4. ESR
5. CRP
6. Rheumatological profile - including a vasculitic screen
7. Aspergillus
8. QuantiFERON gold for TB
9. HIV Testing
10. Arterial blood gases

Imaging Studies

1. Chest X-ray - reticular/ nodular opacities
2. High-resolution CT scan of the thorax - could range from normal to ground glass changes to honey combing in the late stages.

Others

1. ECG
2. Echocardiogram - to look for evidence of pulmonary hypertension

Treatment

General Measures

1. Patient education and advice
2. Smoking cessation
3. Annual vaccinations
4. Healthy diet and exercise
5. Pulmonary rehabilitation
6. Multi-disciplinary involvement - Physiotherapists, occupational therapists, dieticians, psychologists, and social workers

Specific Measures

1. Refer to a respiratory physician and rheumatologist
2. Treatment of condition as appropriate

Case No 10: Consolidation

Introduction

Consolidation is probably the most common condition diagnosed in the Accident and Emergency Department and an easy case for the MRCP exam.

It is essential to assess the severity of the condition post-diagnosis. There are multiple scoring systems to assist in predicting severity and morbidity.

The most common one used is CURB 65:

	Parameters	Score
C	Confusion	1
U	Urea > 7mmol/l	1
R	Respiratory rate > 30br/min	1
Bp - Systolic	</= 90mmHg	1
- Diastolic	</= 60mmHg	
65 yr/>	Age of 65 yrs />	1

CURB 65 Score	Risk group	30-day mortality	Management
0-1	1	1.5%	Home
2	2	9.2%	Likely to need admission
3-5	3	22%	Admit: Treat as severe pneumonia

Other severity scores

1. PSI: Pneumonia severity index
2. PORT: Patient outcomes research teams score
3. APACHE: Acute physiology and chronic health evaluation

Management

Investigations

Blood Tests

1. Full blood count
2. Liver function tests
3. Renal function
4. ESR
5. CRP
6. Blood cultures
7. Arterial blood gases

Imaging Studies

1. Chest X-ray
2. CT Chest
3. Ultrasound chest

Other Investigations

1. Sputum: For microscopy, culture and sensitivity

Pathogen-Specific Tests

1. Urine assays
2. Sputum, serum, and/or urinary antigen tests
3. Immune serologic tests

Invasive Procedures

1. Bronchoscopy
2. Thoracocentesis

Treatment

General Measures

1. Patient education and advice
2. Smoking cessation
3. Annual vaccinations
4. Healthy diet and exercise

Specific Measures

1. Admit patient if severe pneumonia
2. Intravenous antibiotics as per protocol, to convert to oral when stable

Cardiovascular System

Case No 1: Mitral Regurgitation

Mitral regurgitation is one of the most commonly encountered cases in the MRCP PACES exam.

Definition

Mitral Regurgitation is an abnormal reversal of blood flow from the left ventricle to the left atrium.

Aetiology

1. Congenital
2. Mitral valve prolapse
3. Ischaemic heart disease
4. Rheumatic heart disease
5. Myxomatous degeneration of the mitral valve
6. Infective endocarditis
7. Rupture or dysfunction of papillary muscles
8. Other causes: Marfan syndrome, Ehlers Danlos syndrome, dilated cardiomyopathy

Management

Investigations

Blood Tests

1. Full blood count
2. Renal function
3. Liver function
4. ESR
5. CRP
6. Blood cultures - 3 sets in cases of suspected infective endocarditis
7. B-type natriuretic peptide

Imaging Studies

1. Chest X-ray
2. ECG
3. Echocardiogram: Grading the severity of mitral regurgitation:

    Mild: Small central jet of <4cm2, or < 20% of Left atrial area, Vena contracta width of < 0.3cm

    Moderate: Signs of Mitral regurgitation, but not severe

    Severe: Vena contracta width ≥ 0.7cm with large central MR jet (area < 40% of LA)

    or with a wall-impinging jet of any size swirling in LA

    Large flow convergence

    Systolic reversal in pulmonary veins

    Prominent flail MV leaflet or ruptured papillary muscle

Other Investigations

1. Urine - microscopy, culture and sensitivity, microscopic haematuria

Invasive Procedures

1. Cardiac catheterisation with left ventriculography
2. Coronary angiogram

Treatment

General Measures

1. Patient education and advice
2. Promoting a healthy lifestyle - diet/ exercise/ stop smoking
3. Encourage a low sodium diet
4. Advice against recreational drug use in cases of infective endocarditis

Specific Measures

1. Refer to a cardiologist
2. Asymptomatic patients: Regular review with echocardiogram
3. For chronic mitral regurgitation: vasodilators remain the first-line treatment of choice: ACE Inhibitors/ hydralazine
4. Hypertension should be managed aggressively with diuretics
5. Consider digoxin for atrial fibrillation with mitral regurgitation
6. Surgery for symptomatic patients

Indications for surgery

Symptoms	LV EF	LVESD
NYHA II	> 30%	< 55mm
NYHA III-IV	< 30%	> 55mm
Asymptomatic	30 - 60%	≥ 40mm
Asymptomatic with pulmonary hypertension	LV EF > 60% and pulmonary artery systolic pressure > 50 - 60mmHg	
Asymptomatic and the chance for a repair without residual MR is >90%	> 60%	< 40mm

7. Long term follow-up

Case No 2: Mitral Stenosis

Definition

Mitral Stenosis is an obstruction to the inflow into the left ventricle due to a structural abnormality at the level of the mitral valve apparatus.

Aetiology

1. Congenital
2. Rheumatic heart disease
3. Mitral valve calcification
4. Infective endocarditis

Management

Investigations

Blood Tests

1. Full blood count
2. Renal function
3. Liver function
4. ESR
5. CRP
6. Blood cultures - 3 sets in cases of suspected infective endocarditis
7. B-type natriuretic peptide

Imaging Studies

1. Chest X-ray
2. ECG
3. Echocardiogram: Helps to assess severity:

Degree of mitral stenosis	Mean gradient	Mitral valve area
Mild mitral stenosis	< 5mmHg	> $1.5cm^2$
Moderate mitral stenosis	5 - 10mmHg	$1.0 - 1.5cm^2$
Severe mitral stenosis	> 10mmHg	< $1.0cm^2$

Other Investigations

1. Urine - microscopy, culture and sensitivity, microscopic haematuria

Invasive Procedures

1. Cardiac catheterisation with left ventriculography
2. Coronary angiogram

Treatment

General Measures

1. Patient education and advice
2. Promoting a healthy lifestyle - diet/ exercise/ stop smoking
3. Encourage a low sodium diet
4. Advice against recreational drug use in cases of infective endocarditis

Specific Measures

1. Refer to a cardiologist
2. Asymptomatic patients - no treatment necessary - regular monitoring
3. Symptomatic patients:
   a. Medical management: For associated symptoms - angina/ hypertension/ heart failure
   b. Percutaneous mitral valvuloplasty
   c. Surgery - Mitral valve replacement

Case No 3: Aortic Stenosis

Aortic stenosis is another fairly common case in the MRCP PACES Exam.

Definition

Aortic stenosis is an obstruction in the blood flow across the aortic valve.

Aetiology

1. Congenital
2. Bicuspid aortic valve
3. Age-related degeneration of the valve
4. Rheumatic heart disease
5. Associated conditions speeding the process of stenosis- Hypertension/ hyperlipidaemia/ diabetes/ uraemia

Management

Investigations

Blood Tests

1. Full blood count
2. Renal function
3. Liver function

4. ESR
5. CRP
6. Blood cultures - 3 sets in cases of suspected infective endocarditis
7. B-type natriuretic peptide

Imaging Studies

1. Chest X-ray
2. ECG
3. Echocardiogram: Helps to assess severity:

Degree of aortic stenosis	Mean gradient (mmHg)	Aortic valve area (cm^2)
Mild aortic stenosis	< 25	> 1.5
Moderate aortic stenosis	25 - 40	1.0 - 1.5
Severe aortic stenosis	> 40	< 1.0
Critical aortic stenosis	> 70	< 0.6

Other Investigations

1. Urine - microscopy, culture and sensitivity, microscopic haematuria

Invasive Procedures

1. Cardiac catheterisation with left ventriculography
2. Coronary angiogram

Treatment

General Measures

1. Patient education and advice
2. Promoting a healthy lifestyle - diet/ exercise/ stop smoking
3. Encourage a low sodium diet
4. Advice against recreational drug use in cases of infective endocarditis

Specific Measures

1. Refer to a cardiologist
2. Asymptomatic patients - no treatment necessary - regular monitoring
3. Symptomatic patients:
    a. Medical management: For associated symptoms - angina/ hypertension/ heart failure
    b. Percutaneous transcatheter aortic valve replacement
    c. Balloon valvuloplasty
    d. Surgery - Aortic valve replacement

Case No 4: Aortic Regurgitation

Definition

Aortic regurgitation is the incompetence of the aortic valve leading to the diastolic flow of blood from the aorta into the left ventricle.

Aetiology

1. Congenital
2. Rheumatic heart disease
3. Infective endocarditis
4. Degenerative aortic valve disease
5. Hypertension
6. Collagen vascular diseases
7. Others: Syphilitic aortitis, Marfan syndrome, Takayasu's arteritis, ankylosing spondylitis, osteogenesis imperfecta, Bechet's disease, medications like Fenfluramine

Management

Investigations

Blood Tests

1. Full blood count
2. Renal function
3. Liver function

4. ESR
5. CRP
6. Blood cultures - 3 sets in cases of suspected infective endocarditis
7. B-type natriuretic peptide

Imaging Studies

1. Chest X-ray
2. ECG
3. Echocardiogram: Helps assess aortic valve structure, morphology, and regurgitant jet severity.

Other Investigations

1. Urine - microscopy/ culture/ sensitivity, microscopic haematuria

Invasive Procedures

1. Cardiac catheterisation with left ventriculography
2. Coronary angiogram

Treatment

General Measures

1. Patient education and advice
2. Promoting a healthy lifestyle - diet/ exercise/ stop smoking
3. Encourage a low sodium diet
4. Advice against recreational drug use in cases of infective endocarditis

Specific Measures

1. Refer to a cardiologist
2. Asymptomatic patients - regular monitoring
3. Symptomatic patients:
    a. Medical management:
        i. For associated symptoms - angina/ hypertension/ heart failure
        ii. Vasodilators - ACE Inhibitors/ angiotensin receptor blockers (ARBs)/ Nifedipine/ Hydralazine
    b. Percutaneous transcatheter aortic valve replacement
    c. Surgery - Aortic valve replacement

Indications for surgery in chronic aortic regurgitation

Symptoms	Ejection fraction	Additional findings
Present (NYHA II-IV)	Any	
Absent	> 50%	Abnormal exercise test, severe LV dilatation (systolic ventricular diameter >55mm)
Absent	<=50%	
Cardiac surgery for other causes (i.e., CAD, other valvular diseases, ascending aortic aneurysm)		

Case No 5: Valve Replacements

Introduction

Patients with mitral and aortic valve replacements are commonly found in the MRCP PACES exam.

Types of Valves

1. Mechanical valves
2. Bioprosthetic/ tissue valves

Indications for Valve Replacement

1. Mitral or Aortic incompetence
2. Mitral or aortic stenosis

	Tissue valves	Mechanical valves
Lifetime of valve	10 - 15 years	> 15 years
Anticoagulation	Not required	Lifetime anticoagulation

Management

Investigations

Blood Tests

1. Full blood count
2. Renal function
3. Liver function
4. ESR
5. CRP
6. B-type natriuretic peptide
7. Troponin if there is suspected ischaemic heart disease

Imaging Studies

1. Chest X-ray
2. ECG
3. Echocardiogram: Peri membranous/ supracristal/ muscular/ atrioventricular septal defects (AVSDs)

Other Investigations

1. Urine - microscopy, culture and sensitivity, microscopic haematuria

Invasive Procedures

1. Cardiac catheterisation with left ventriculography
2. Coronary angiogram

Treatment

General Measures

1. Patient education and advice
2. Promoting a healthy lifestyle - diet/ exercise/ stop smoking
3. Encourage a low sodium diet
4. Advice against recreational drug use in cases of infective endocarditis

Specific Measures

1. Refer to a cardiologist
2. Asymptomatic patients - regular monitoring

Case No 6: Combined Valve Lesions

Types of Combined Valve Lesions

1. Mitral and aortic regurgitation
2. Mitral and aortic stenosis
3. Mitral stenosis and aortic regurgitation
4. Aortic stenosis and mitral regurgitation

Common Causes for Combined Valve Lesions

1. Rheumatic heart disease
2. Degenerative valvular disease
3. Other associated conditions: Hypertension, diabetes, dyslipidaemia, connective tissue disorders, infective endocarditis, cardiomyopathies

Management

Investigations

Blood Tests

1. Full blood count
2. Renal function
3. Liver function
4. ESR
5. CRP
6. B-type natriuretic peptide

7. Troponin if the patient has suspected Ischaemic heart disease

Imaging Studies

1. Chest X-ray
2. ECG
3. Echocardiogram: To determine valve lesion and severity

Other Investigations

1. Urine - microscopy, culture and sensitivity, microscopic haematuria

Invasive Procedures

1. Cardiac catheterisation with left ventriculography
2. Coronary angiogram

Treatment

General Measures

1. Patient education and advice
2. Promoting a healthy lifestyle - diet/ exercise/ stop smoking
3. Encourage a low sodium diet
4. Advice against recreational drug use in cases of infective endocarditis

Specific Measures

1. Refer to a cardiologist
2. Asymptomatic patients - regular monitoring

Case No 7: Ventricular Septal Defect

Definition

A ventricular septal defect (VSD) is a defect in the ventricular septum, resulting in communication between the two ventricular cavities.

Aetiology

1. Genetic causes
2. Maternal diabetes

Management

Investigations

Blood Tests

1. Full blood count
2. Renal function
3. Liver function
4. ESR
5. CRP
6. B-type natriuretic peptide
7. Troponin if the patient has suspected Ischaemic heart disease

Imaging Studies

1. Chest X-ray
2. ECG
3. Echocardiogram: Peri membranous/ supracristal/ muscular/ AVSDs
4. Cardiac MRI

Other Investigations

1. Urine - microscopy, culture and sensitivity, microscopic haematuria

Invasive Procedures

1. Cardiac catheterisation with left ventriculography
2. Coronary angiogram

Treatment

General Measures

1. Patient education and advice
2. Promoting a healthy lifestyle - diet/ exercise/ stop smoking
3. Encourage a low sodium diet
4. Advice against recreational drug use in cases of infective endocarditis

Specific Measures

1. Refer to a cardiologist
2. Asymptomatic patients - regular monitoring
3. Medical management of congestive heart failure
4. Surgical intervention in symptomatic patients
5. Long term monitoring

Case No 8: Fallot's Tetralogy

Components

1. Ventricular septal defect
2. Overriding aorta
3. Pulmonary stenosis
4. Right ventricular hypertrophy

Blalock Taussig shunt

- Anastomosis between the subclavian artery and pulmonary artery

Modified Blalock Taussig Shunt

- Anastomosis between the subclavian artery and pulmonary artery, with a graft

Management

Investigations

Blood Tests

1. Full blood count
2. Renal function
3. Liver function
4. ESR
5. CRP

6. B-type natriuretic peptide
7. Troponin if the patient has suspected ischaemic heart disease
8. Arterial blood gases

Imaging Studies

1. Chest X-ray
2. ECG
3. Echocardiogram
4. Cardiac MRI

Other Investigations

1. Urine - microscopy, culture and sensitivity, microscopic haematuria

Invasive Procedures

1. Cardiac catheterisation with left ventriculography
2. Coronary angiogram

Treatment

General Measures

1. Patient education and advice
2. Promoting a healthy lifestyle - diet/ exercise/ stop smoking
3. Encourage a low sodium diet
4. Advice against recreational drug use in cases of infective endocarditis

Specific measures

1. Refer to a cardiologist
2. Asymptomatic patients - regular monitoring
3. Referral to the cardiothoracic surgeons
4. Long term monitoring
5. Management of associated complications

Case No 9: Tricuspid/Pulmonary Regurgitation

Tricuspid Regurgitation

Aetiology

1. Ebstein's anomaly
2. Rheumatic fever
3. Carcinoid tumours
4. Any cause of pulmonary hypertension
5. Connective tissue diseases like Marfan Syndrome
6. Rheumatoid arthritis
7. Injury
8. Radiation therapy

Pulmonary Regurgitation

Aetiology

1. Pulmonary hypertension
2. Rheumatic heart disease
3. Infective endocarditis
4. Carcinoid syndrome
5. Tetralogy of Fallot

Management

Investigations

Blood Tests

1. Full blood count
2. Renal function
3. Liver function
4. ESR
5. CRP
6. B-type natriuretic peptide
7. Troponin if the patient has suspected ischaemic heart disease
8. Arterial blood gases

Imaging Studies

1. Chest X-ray
2. ECG
3. Echocardiogram
4. Cardiac MRI

Other Investigations

1. Urine - microscopy, culture and sensitivity, microscopic haematuria

Invasive Procedures

1. Cardiac catheterisation with left ventriculography
2. Coronary angiogram

Treatment

General Measures

1. Patient education and advice
2. Promoting a healthy lifestyle - diet/ exercise/ stop smoking
3. Encourage a low sodium diet
4. Advice against recreational drug use in cases of infective endocarditis

Specific Measures

1. Refer to a cardiologist
2. Asymptomatic patients - regular monitoring
3. Referral to the cardiothoracic surgeons when appropriate
4. Long term monitoring
5. Management of associated complications

Case No 10: Rarer Cases

A] Dextrocardia

Points to remember

i.   Congenital problem with the heart situated on the right side of the body

ii. It may be associated with other congenital cardiac defects, including endocardial cushion defects, double outlet right ventricle, etc.

iii. Kartagener's syndrome: Chronic sinusitis, situs inversus and primary ciliary dyskinesia

B] Patent Ductus Arteriosus

Points to remember

i.   A congenital disorder resulting in the failure of closure of the ductus arteriosus leading to communication between the descending thoracic aorta and the pulmonary artery

ii. Associated with chromosomal abnormalities like Down's syndrome, congenital rubella and pre-term delivery

iii. Treatment options could be nonsurgical with prostaglandins and non-steroidal anti-inflammatory drugs (NSAIDs) and surgical in the form of ligation procedures

C] Coarctation of Aorta

Points to remember

i.   A congenital disorder resulting in narrowing of the aorta is commonly just distal to the origin of the left subclavian artery

ii. Types:

   a.   Pre-ductal coarctation - Associated with Turner syndrome

   b.   Ductal coarctation

   c.   Post ductal coarctation - most commonly seen in adults

D] Hypertrophic Cardiomyopathy

Aetiology

A genetic disorder causes myocardial hypertrophy leading to one of the most common causes of sudden cardiac death.

Management

Investigations

Blood Tests

1.   Full blood count
2.   Renal function
3.   Liver function
4.   ESR
5.   CRP
6.   B-type natriuretic peptide
7.   Troponin if the patient has suspected ischaemic heart disease
8.   Arterial blood gases

Imaging Studies
1. Chest X-ray
2. ECG
3. Echocardiogram
4. Cardiac MRI

Other Investigations
1. Urine - microscopy, culture and sensitivity, microscopic haematuria

Treatment

General Measures

1. Patient education and advice
2. Promoting a healthy lifestyle - diet/ exercise/ stop smoking
3. Encourage a low sodium diet
4. Advice against recreational drug use in cases of infective endocarditis

Specific Measures
1. Refer to a cardiologist
2. Asymptomatic patients - regular monitoring

Central Nervous System

Case No 1: Cerebellar Syndrome

Aetiology

Common Causes

1. Alcoholic cerebellar degeneration
2. Posterior fossa tumours
3. Multiple sclerosis
4. Paraneoplastic cerebellar degeneration
5. Cerebellar stroke

Other Causes

1. Rarer - Friedreich's ataxia, Wilson's disease
2. Hypothyroidism
3. Infections: Meningitis/ abscess
4. Drugs: Phenytoin, barbiturates

Management

Investigations

Blood Tests

1. Full blood count
2. Renal function
3. Liver function
4. ESR
5. CRP

6. Autoimmune screen, serum caeruloplasmin
7. Vitamin B12/ Folic acid levels
8. Tumour markers if malignancy suspected
9. Thyroid function tests
10. Fasting blood glucose
11. Lipids
12. Serum protein electrophoresis, immunoglobulins
13. Drug levels
14. Blood cultures

Imaging Studies

1. Chest X-ray
2. ECG
3. CT brain
4. MRI brain
5. Electroencephalogram (EEG)

Other Investigations

1. Urine - microscopy, culture and sensitivity, microscopic haematuria
2. Lumbar puncture - if suspected meningitis

Treatment

General Measures

1. Patient education and advice
2. Promoting a healthy lifestyle - diet/ exercise/ stop smoking
3. Look at reversible causes - Cutting down on alcohol intake, advise against recreational drug use

Specific Measures

1. Refer to a neurologist
2. Refer to an oncologist if malignancy suspected
3. Multi-disciplinary team involvement - Alcohol and drug team referral, social services, physiotherapy, occupational therapy, speech and language therapy
4. Treatment of any underlying cause

Case No 2: Peripheral Neuropathy

Aetiology

Sensory Neuropathy

1. Paraneoplastic/ autoimmune neuropathy
2. Diabetic neuropathy
3. Toxins (Chemotherapy drugs, chloroquine, metronidazole)
4. HIV
5. Sjogren's syndrome

Motor Neuropathy

1. Porphyria
2. Chronic Inflammatory demyelinating polyneuropathy
3. Hypothyroidism
4. Toxins (Dapsone, Vincristine, Amiodarone)
5. Guillain-Barre syndrome
6. Dysproteinaemias
7. Diphtheria

Sensorimotor Neuropathy

1. Alcoholic neuropathy
2. Diabetic neuropathy
3. Hereditary sensorimotor neuropathy

4. Vitamin deficiencies - B12/ B1/ E
5. Paraneoplastic neuropathy
6. Connective tissue diseases
7. Toxins (metals, Nitrofurantoin, Chemotherapy drugs)

Management

Investigations

Blood Tests

1. Full blood count
2. Renal function
3. Liver function
4. ESR
5. CRP
6. Autoimmune screen, serum caeruloplasmin
7. Vitamin B12/ Folic acid levels
8. Tumour markers if malignancy suspected
9. Thyroid function tests
10. Fasting blood glucose and HbA1C
11. Lipids
12. Serum protein electrophoresis, immunoglobulins
13. Drug levels
14. Blood cultures

Imaging Studies

1. Chest X-ray
2. ECG
3. CT chest/ abdomen /pelvis - if suspected malignancy
4. Skeletal survey

Other Investigations

1. Urine - microscopy, culture and sensitivity
2. Electromyography
3. Nerve conduction studies
4. Nerve biopsy
5. Lumbar puncture

Treatment

General Measures

1. Patient education and advice
2. Promoting a healthy lifestyle - diet/ exercise/ stop smoking
3. Look at reversible causes - Cutting down on alcohol intake, advice against recreational drug use

Specific Measures

1. Refer to a neurologist
2. Refer to an oncologist if malignancy suspected
3. Multi-disciplinary team involvement - Alcohol and drug team referral, social services, physiotherapy, occupational therapy, speech and language therapy
4. Treatment of any underlying cause

Case No 3: Hemiplegia

Aetiology

Ischaemic Stroke

1. Thrombosis - arterial or venous
2. Embolism
3. Systemic hypoperfusion - shock

Haemorrhagic Stroke

1. Intraparenchymal haemorrhage
2. Subdural haematoma
3. Subarachnoid haemorrhage

Management

Investigations

Blood Tests

1. Full blood count
2. Renal function
3. Liver function
4. ESR
5. CRP
6. Autoimmune screen, serum ceruloplasmin
7. Vitamin B12/ Folic acid levels
8. Vasculitic screen

9. Thyroid function tests
10. Fasting blood glucose and HbA1C
11. Lipids
12. Serum protein electrophoresis, immunoglobulins
13. Homocysteine level
14. Cardiac biomarkers
15. Drug levels
16. Blood cultures

Imaging Studies

1. CT + CTA brain
2. MRI + MRA + MRV brain
3. Carotid dopplers
4. Echocardiogram
5. Chest X-ray
6. ECG

Other Investigations

1. Lumbar puncture

Treatment

General Measures

1. Patient education and advice
2. Promoting a healthy lifestyle - diet/ exercise/ stop smoking
3. Look at reversible causes - Cutting down on alcohol intake, advice against recreational drug use

Specific Measures

1. Refer to a neurologist/ stroke physician
2. Acute management includes patient stabilisation and fibrinolysis based on the National Institutes of Health Stroke Scale (NIHSS)
3. Reperfusion therapy: Thrombolysis with tenecteplase/ alteplase
4. Neurointervention: Endovascular thrombectomy
5. Antiplatelet therapy with Aspirin/ Dipyridamole
6. Managing secondary risk factors - Hypertension/ diabetes/ hypercholesterolaemia
7. Monitor for seizures
8. Multi-disciplinary team involvement - Physiotherapy, occupational therapy, speech and language therapy, social services
9. Vascular surgery referral in case of severe carotid artery stenosis
10. Cardiology referral in case of atrial fibrillation/ valvular disease/ heart failure

Other points to remember

Stroke Classification (Bamford classification)

Total Anterior Circulation Stroke (TACS)

All three of the following:

1. Unilateral weakness (and/or sensory deficit) of face, arm and leg
2. Homonymous hemianopia
3. Higher cerebral dysfunction (dysphasia, visuospatial disorder)

Partial Anterior Circulation Stroke (PACS)

Two of the following:

1. Unilateral weakness (and/or sensory deficit) of face, arm and leg
2. Homonymous hemianopia
3. Higher cerebral dysfunction (dysphasia, visuospatial disorder)

Posterior Circulation Syndrome (POCS)

One of the following:

1. Cerebellar or brainstem syndromes
2. Loss of consciousness
3. Isolated homonymous hemianopia

Lacunar Syndrome (LACS)

One of the following:

1. Unilateral weakness (and/or sensory deficit) of face and arm, arm and leg or all three.
2. Pure sensory stroke.
3. Ataxic hemiparesis.

Case No 4: Charcot-Marie-Tooth Disease

Aetiology

Also known as "hereditary sensory motor neuropathy"

Types
CMT 1: Demyelinating type - impairs nerve conduction velocity

CMT 2: Axonal type

CMT 3: Dejerine-Sottas disease - does not impair nerve conduction velocity

Others

Management

Investigations

Routine bloods - usually within normal limits

Genetic tests
Imaging Studies
1. MRI lower limbs

Others
1. Electromyography
2. Nerve conduction studies

Treatment

General Measures

1. Patient education and advice
2. Promoting a healthy lifestyle - diet/ exercise/ stop smoking
3. Look at reversible causes - Cutting down on alcohol intake, advice against recreational drug use

Specific Measures

1. Refer to a neurologist
2. Multi-disciplinary team involvement - Physiotherapy, occupational therapy, speech and language therapy, social services
3. Referral to orthopaedic surgeons for osteotomies/ joint stabilisation procedures

Case No 5: Parkinson's Disease

Aetiology

1. Idiopathic
2. Environmental factors: Exposure to pesticides, herbicides, industrial plants or quarries
3. MPTP injection - 1-methyl-4-phenyl-1,2,3,6-tetrahydropyridine
4. Genetic factors
5. Hypoxic brain injury
6. Oxidation hypothesis – due to dopamine's oxidative metabolism

Management

Investigations

Blood Tests

1. Full blood count
2. Renal function
3. Liver function
4. ESR
5. CRP
6. Autoimmune screen, serum ceruloplasmin
7. Vitamin B12/ Folic acid levels
8. Vasculitic screen
9. Thyroid function tests

10. Fasting blood glucose and HbA1C
11. Lipids
12. Serum protein electrophoresis, immunoglobulins
13. Homocysteine level
14. Cardiac biomarkers
15. Drug levels
16. Blood cultures

Imaging Studies
1. CT + CTA brain
2. MRI + MRA + MRV brain
3. Carotid dopplers
4. Echocardiogram
5. Chest X-ray
6. ECG

Other Investigations
1. Lumbar puncture

Treatment

General Measures

1. Patient education and advice
2. Promoting a healthy lifestyle - diet/ exercise/ stop smoking
3. Look for reversible causes - Cutting down on alcohol intake, advice against recreational drug use

Specific Measures

1. Refer to a neurologist
2. Medications:
   a. Dopamine agonists: Levodopa/ Carbidopa, Apomorphine, Pramipexole, Ropinirole, Amantadine, Rotigotine
   b. Anticholinergic drugs: Benztropine
   c. MAO B Inhibitors: Selegiline, Rasagiline
   d. Acetyl Cholinesterase inhibitors: Donepezil, Rivastigmine, Galantamine
   e. N Methyl D Aspartate receptor antagonist: Memantine
   f. Catechol O Methyl Transferase inhibitors: Entacapone, Tolcapone
3. Multi-disciplinary team involvement: Physiotherapist, occupational therapy, neuropsychologist, social services, dietician, etc
4. Newer treatment: Deep brain stimulation, thalamotomy, pallidotomy
5. Involvement of the neuro-rehabilitation team in advanced cases

Case No 6: Myotonic Dystrophy

Aetiology

There are two types of Myotonic Dystrophy. Both are autosomal dominant. They are caused by a mutation called "anticipation, " meaning that the same three nucleotide sequence repeats several times.

1. Type 1: Caused by a mutation in the DMPK gene, also known as Steinert disease, severe congenital form.
2. Type 2: Caused by mutations in the CMBP gene, also known as proximal myotonic myopathy, rarer and manifests with milder signs and symptoms.

Management

Investigations

Blood Tests

1. Full blood count
2. Renal function
3. Liver function
4. ESR
5. CRP
6. Autoimmune screen, serum ceruloplasmin
7. Vitamin B12/ Folic acid levels

8. Vasculitic screen
9. Thyroid function tests
10. Fasting blood glucose and HbA1C
11. Lipids
12. Serum protein electrophoresis, immunoglobulins
13. Homocysteine level
14. Cardiac biomarkers
15. Drug levels
16. Blood cultures

Imaging Studies

1. CT + CTA brain
2. MRI + MRA + MRV brain
3. Carotid dopplers
4. Echocardiogram
5. Chest X-ray
6. ECG

Other Investigations

1. Lumbar puncture

Treatment

General Measures

1. Patient education and advice
2. Promoting a healthy lifestyle - diet/ exercise/ stop smoking
3. Look at reversible causes - Cutting down on alcohol intake, advice against recreational drug use

Specific Measures

1. Multi-disciplinary approach - Neurology, cardiology, ophthalmology, endocrinology, rheumatology
2. Physiotherapist, occupational therapy, neuropsychologist, social services, dietician, speech and language therapy, etc
3. Symptomatic treatment
4. Caution with a general anaesthetic
5. Sleep studies and consideration of non-invasive ventilation
6. Pacemaker insertion

Case No 7: Visual Field Defects

Aetiology

1. Cerebrovascular accident
2. Tumours:
   a. Craniopharyngioma
   b. Pituitary tumour
   c. Glioma
   d. Meningioma
3. Hydrocephalus
4. Drugs: E.g. Vigabatrin
5. Ocular causes: Glaucoma, macular degeneration, retinitis pigmentosa, optic neuritis, Leber's optic atrophy, ischaemic optic neuropathy
6. Demyelination
7. Vascular causes
8. Others: Migraine, vasculitis, nutritional deficiencies, toxins

Management

Investigations

Blood Tests

1. Full blood count
2. Renal function
3. Liver function

4. ESR
5. CRP
6. Autoimmune screen, serum caeruloplasmin
7. Vitamin B12/ Folic acid levels
8. Vasculitic screen
9. Thyroid function tests
10. Fasting blood glucose and HbA1C
11. Lipids
12. Serum protein electrophoresis, immunoglobulins
13. Homocysteine level
14. Cardiac biomarkers
15. Drug levels
16. Blood cultures

Imaging Studies
1. CT + CTA brain
2. MRI + MRA + MRV brain
3. Carotid dopplers
4. Echocardiogram
5. Chest X-ray
6. ECG
7. Perimetry

Other Investigations
1. Lumbar puncture

Treatment

General Measures

1. Patient education and advice
2. Promoting a healthy lifestyle - diet/ exercise/ stop smoking
3. Look at reversible causes - Cutting down on alcohol intake, advice against recreational drug use

Specific Measures

1. Refer to a neurologist/ stroke physician
2. Referral to an ophthalmologist for ocular causes
3. Managing secondary risk factors - Hypertension/ diabetes/ hypercholesterolaemia
4. Multi-disciplinary team involvement - Physiotherapy, occupational therapy, speech and language therapy, social services
5. Treatment of any underlying cause

Case No 8: Spastic Paraparesis

Aetiology

1. Hereditary spastic paraplegia
2. Hereditary spinocerebellar degeneration - Friedrich's ataxia
3. Multiple sclerosis
4. Cervical spondylosis
5. Subacute combined degeneration of the cord
6. Spinal tumours - meningioma
7. Spinal arteriovenous shunts
8. Infections: Tropical spastic paraparesis, Lyme disease, syphilis, AIDS

Management

Investigations

Blood Tests

1. Full blood count
2. Renal function
3. Liver function
4. ESR, CRP
5. Fasting blood glucose and HbA1C
6. Lipids
7. Vitamin B12 and caeruloplasmin levels

8. Blood cultures
9. Screen for infections - HIV, Lyme disease, syphilis
10. Genetic testing

Imaging Studies

1. CT brain
2. MRI brain and spinal cord
3. Chest X-ray
4. ECG

Other Investigations

1. Lumbar puncture

Treatment

General Measures

1. Patient education and advice
2. Promoting a healthy lifestyle - diet/ exercise/ stop smoking
3. Consider reversible causes - Cutting down on alcohol intake, advice against recreational drug use

Specific Measures

1. Refer to a neurologist/ stroke physician
2. Managing secondary risk factors - Hypertension/ diabetes/ hypercholesterolaemia
3. Multi-disciplinary team involvement - Physiotherapy, occupational therapy, speech and language therapy, social services
4. Treatment of any underlying cause

Case No 9: Facial Nerve Palsy

Aetiology

1. Bell's palsy
2. Infection - Herpes zoster - Ramsay Hunt syndrome, Lyme disease
3. Trauma - Fractures of the temporal bone
4. Tumours - Facial neuromas, congenital cholesteatomas, haemangiomas, acoustic neuromas and metastases
5. Metabolic - Diabetes, hyperthyroidism, porphyria, vitamin A deficiency
6. Iatrogenic - Mandibular surgery, post immunisation, parotid surgery, post-tonsillectomy and adenoidectomy
7. Others - Myasthenia gravis, autoimmune conditions, sarcoidosis, amyloidosis
8. Cerebrovascular accident

Management

Investigations

Blood Tests

1. Full blood count
2. Renal function
3. Liver function

4. ESR, CRP
5. Fasting blood glucose and HbA1C
6. Lipids
7. Vitamin B12 and caeruloplasmin levels
8. Thyroid function tests
9. Blood cultures
10. Screen for infections - Herpes zoster, Lyme disease
11. Autoimmune screen
12. Acetylcholine receptor antibodies, serum ACE levels, etc

Imaging Studies
1. CT brain
2. MRI brain
3. Facial bones X-ray

Other Investigations
1. Lumbar puncture
2. Electrophysiology

Treatment

General Measures

1. Patient education and advice
2. Promoting a healthy lifestyle - diet/ exercise/ stop smoking
3. Look at reversible causes - Cutting down on alcohol intake, advice against recreational drug use

Specific Measures

1. Refer to a neurologist/ stroke physician
2. Managing secondary risk factors - Hypertension/ diabetes/ hypercholesterolaemia
3. Treatment for a cerebrovascular accident, if appropriate for central facial nerve palsy
4. Multi-disciplinary team involvement – Physiotherapy, occupational therapy, speech and language therapy, social services
5. Referral to surgery if appropriate
6. Eye protection and management of drooling
7. Treatment of any underlying cause

Case No 10: Other Cases

A] Motor Neurone Disease

Aetiology

Mainly unknown - possible sporadic

Classification

1. Amyotrophic lateral sclerosis (Lou Gehrig's disease) - Both upper motor neurone (UMN) and lower motor neurone (LMN) signs
2. Primary lateral sclerosis - Mainly UMN signs
3. Progressive muscular atrophy - Mainly LMN signs
4. Progressive bulbar palsy - Mainly LMN bulbar palsy - poor prognosis
5. Pseudobulbar palsy - Mainly UMN bulbar involvement

Management

Investigations

Blood Tests

1. Full blood count
2. Renal function
3. Liver function
4. ESR

5. CRP
6. Autoimmune screen, serum caeruloplasmin
7. Vitamin B12/ Folic acid levels
8. Vasculitic screen
9. Thyroid function tests
10. Fasting blood glucose and HbA1C
11. Lipids
12. Serum protein electrophoresis, immunoglobulins
13. Homocysteine level
14. Cardiac biomarkers
15. Drug levels
16. Blood cultures

Imaging

1. CT + CTA brain
2. MRI + MRA + MRV brain

Other tests

1. Lumbar puncture
2. Nerve conduction tests
3. Electromyographic studies

Treatment

General Measures

1. Patient education and advice
2. Promoting a healthy lifestyle - diet/ exercise/ stop smoking
3. Look at reversible causes - Cutting down on alcohol intake, advice against recreational drug use

Specific Measures

1. Refer to a neurologist
2. Multi-disciplinary approach: Physiotherapists, occupational therapists, social workers, psychologists, speech and language therapists, and dieticians
3. Riluzole - may be tried - evidence exists that it may prolong life by 2 - 3 months but does not improve symptoms
4. Symptomatic management:
   a. Muscle cramps/ spasticity
   b. Swallowing difficulties
   c. Drooling
   d. Communication difficulties
   e. Pain relief
   f. Treatment of infections
   g. Shortness of breath - may get symptomatic relief with non-invasive ventilation
5. Advanced health directive
6. Palliative care referral

B] Mononeuropathies:

Ulnar Nerve Palsy/ Radial Nerve Palsy/ Carpal Tunnel Syndrome/ Common Peroneal Nerve Palsy

Aetiology

1. Injury
2. Compressive lesions
3. Systemic conditions: Diabetes, rheumatoid arthritis, vasculitis, amyloidosis, hypothyroidism, acromegaly

4. Vitamin deficiencies
5. Entrapment neuropathy

Management

Investigations

Blood Tests

1. Full blood count
2. Renal function
3. Liver function
4. ESR
5. CRP
6. Autoimmune screen, serum caeruloplasmin
7. Vitamin B12/ Folic acid levels
8. Tumour markers if malignancy suspected
9. Thyroid function tests
10. Fasting blood glucose and HbA1C
11. Lipids
12. Serum protein electrophoresis, immunoglobulins
13. Drug levels
14. Blood cultures

Imaging Studies

1. Chest X-ray
2. ECG
3. CT chest/ abdomen /pelvis - if suspected malignancy
4. Skeletal survey

Other investigations

1. Electromyography
2. Nerve conduction studies
3. Nerve biopsy
4. Lumbar puncture

Treatment

General Measures

1. Patient education and advice
2. Promoting a healthy lifestyle - diet/ exercise/ stop smoking
3. Look at reversible causes - Cutting down on alcohol intake, advice against recreational drug use

Specific Measures

1. Refer to a neurologist
2. Refer to an oncologist if malignancy suspected
3. Refer to the orthopaedic team if trauma/ entrapment/ compression is suspected
4. Multi-disciplinary team involvement - Alcohol and drug team referral, social services, physiotherapy, occupational therapy, speech and language therapy
5. Treatment of any underlying cause

C] Friedreich's Ataxia

Aetiology

Autosomal recessive condition with a genetic focus on Chromosome 9

Management

Investigations

Blood Tests

1. Full blood count
2. Renal function
3. Liver function
4. ESR
5. CRP
6. Autoimmune screen, serum ceruloplasmin
7. Vitamin B12/ Folic acid levels
8. Thyroid function tests
9. Fasting blood glucose
10. Lipids
11. Genetic test

Imaging Studies

1. CT brain
2. MRI brain
3. Visual evoked potentials

Others Investigations

1. ECG
2. Echocardiography
3. Brainstem auditory evoked responses

Treatment

General Measures

1. Patient education and advice

2. Promoting a healthy lifestyle - diet/ exercise/ stop smoking
3. Look at other aspects of lifestyle - Cutting down on alcohol intake, advice against recreational drug use

Specific Measures

1. Multi-disciplinary approach - Neurology, Cardiology, Surgeons
2. Physiotherapist, Occupational Therapy, Neuropsychologist, Social Services, Dietician, Speech and Language Therapy, etc
3. Symptomatic treatment
4. Genetic counselling

D] Horner's Syndrome

Aetiology

1. First-order neuron lesions:
- Demyelinating disease
- Pituitary tumour
- Cerebrovascular accident
- Basal meningitis
- Syringomyelia

2. Second-order neuron lesions:
- Pancoast's tumour
- Cervical rib
- Central venous cannulation
- Lymphadenopathy

3. Third-order neuron lesions:

- Internal carotid artery dissection
- Carotid cavernous fistula
- Migraine
- Herpes zoster

Treatment

General Measures

1. Patient education and advice
2. Promoting a healthy lifestyle - diet/ exercise/ stop smoking
3. Look at other aspects of lifestyle - Cutting down on alcohol intake, advice against recreational drug use

Specific Measures

1. Treatment of any underlying cause
2. Refer to a neurologist/ oncologist as appropriate
3. Refer to a neuro-ophthalmologist and surgeon as appropriate

Rarer Cases:

E] Polio

Aetiology

Caused by poliovirus member of the genus enterovirus of the picornavirus family. It belongs to a group of RNA viruses. It is spread by the faecal-oral route and by aerosol droplets.

Points to remember

1. It causes a flaccid paralysis due to the involvement of the anterior horn motor neurons in the spinal cord and brain stem

2. Most commonly occurs in the paediatric population

3. Non-paralytic poliomyelitis may cause a minor illness with complete recovery though few cases may progress to the paralytic type

4. Paralytic poliomyelitis causes flaccid paralysis with initially brisk reflexes, which become absent later.

5. Post-polio syndrome is rarely life-threatening but occurs in patients who have survived an acute attack and years after recovery, with weakening in muscles previously affected by the polio infection

F] Cervical Myelopathy

Aetiology

1. Degenerative disease of the cervical spine
2. Central disc prolapsed
3. Tumours
4. Infection

Points to remember

1. Insidious onset

2. Spastic gait with brisk reflexes in the lower limbs and upper limbs below the level of the lesion with extensor plantars

3. Positive Lhermitte's sign: Neck extension leading to a generalised electric shock-like sensation

4. Positive Hoffman sign: Forced flexion of the distal

interphalangeal joint of the middle finger leading to a reflex contraction of the thumb and index fingers, indicating a UMN lesion

G] Cerebello-Pontine Angle Lesion

Aetiology

1. Commonest - Vestibular schwannomas or acoustic neuromas
2. Lipomas
3. Haemangiomas and other vascular malformations
4. Meningiomas
5. Facial or lower cranial nerve schwannomas
6. Cholesteatomas
7. Primary or metastatic lesion

Points to remember

1. Involvement of cranial nerves V, VII, VIII
2. Sensorineural hearing loss/ deafness with altered gait and vertigo may be present

H] Absent Ankle Jerks with Extensor Plantars

Aetiology

1. Subacute combined degeneration of the spinal cord
2. Motor neuron disease
3. Tabes dorsalis
4. Friedreich's ataxia
5. Cerebrovascular accident with diabetes
6. Cauda equina lesion

I] Cranial Nerve Lesions

Common causes

1. Bell's palsy - described above
2. Visual field defects - described above
3. Ophthalmoplegia

Brief Clinical Consultations: Rheumatology

Case No 1. Rheumatoid Arthritis

Aetiology

Chronic systemic inflammatory disease of no known recognised aetiology, causing a generalised autoimmune reaction leading to articular and extra-articular manifestations.

Important points to remember

- Symmetrical polyarthritis affecting hands and feet
- Look for extra-articular manifestations
- Do not forget cervical spine examination

Management

Investigations

Blood Tests

1. Full blood count
2. Urea and electrolytes
3. Liver function tests
4. Erythrocyte sedimentation rate
5. Rheumatoid factor assay
6. C-Reactive protein
7. Anti-nuclear antibody assay
8. Anti-cyclic – citrullinated peptide assay
9. Anti-mutated citrullinated vimentin assay

Imaging Studies

1. Plain X-rays of hands, wrists, elbows, shoulders, hips, knees, feet, cervical spine
2. MRI of the cervical spine, if indicated
3. Ultrasonography for effusions
4. CT of affected joints when indicated

Other Investigations

1. Joint aspiration
2. Investigations for extra-articular manifestations as appropriate

Treatment

General Measures

1. Patient education and advice
2. Promoting a healthy lifestyle - diet/ exercise/ stop smoking
3. Look at other aspects of lifestyle - Cutting down on alcohol intake, advice against recreational drug use

Specific Measures

1. Refer to a rheumatologist
2. Non-pharmacologic therapies:
    a. Physiotherapy
    b. Occupational therapy
    c. Education for joint protection and preservation
    d. Orthotics and splints
    e. Heat and cold therapy
    f. Hydrotherapy
    g. Adaptive equipment

3. Pharmacologic therapy:
   a. Non-biologic disease-modifying antirheumatic drugs (DMARDS) are first-line treatment options: Methotrexate, Hydroxychloroquine, Sulphasalazine, Leflunomide, Azathioprine, Gold, D-Penicillamine, Cyclosporine
   b. Biologic DMARDS: TNF inhibitors: Etanercept, Infliximab, Adalimumab, Certolizumab, Golimumab
   c. Other biologic DMARDS: Rituximab (Anti CD20), Anakinra (Anti IL 1), Abatacept (Selective co-stimulation modulator – inhibits co-stimulation of T Cells), Tocilizumab (Anti IL 6), Tofacitinib (Anti Janus kinase 3)
   d. Other drugs: NSAIDs, Corticosteroids, other analgesics
4. Surgical treatments: Synovectomy, tendon realignment, tenosynovectomy, arthrodesis and reconstructive surgery or arthroplasty

Case No 2: Psoriatic Arthropathy

Aetiology

Psoriatic Arthropathy is a seronegative arthritis commonly seen with psoriasis, which may or may not precede the skin manifestations

Types of psoriatic arthritis

a. Symmetrical polyarthritis
b. Distal interphalangeal joint arthropathy
c. Asymmetrical oligoarthritis
d. Spondylitis without sacroiliitis
e. Arthritis mutilans

Management

Investigations

Blood Tests

1. Full blood count
2. Urea and electrolytes
3. Liver function tests
4. Erythrocyte sedimentation rate
5. Rheumatoid factor assay
6. C-reactive protein
7. Anti-nuclear antibody assay
8. Serum immunoglobulin levels

9. Serum urate level
10. HLA B27, HLA B7 and HLA DR4 levels

Imaging Studies
1. Plain X-rays of hands, wrists, elbows, shoulders, hips, knees, feet, spine
2. MRI of the spine, if indicated
3. Ultrasonography for effusions
4. CT of affected joints when indicated

Other Investigations
1. Joint aspiration
2. Investigations for extra-articular manifestations as appropriate.

Treatment

General Measures
1. Patient education and advice
2. Promoting a healthy lifestyle - diet/ exercise/ stop smoking
3. Look at other aspects of lifestyle - Cutting down on alcohol intake, advice against recreational drug use

Specific Measures
1. Refer to a rheumatologist
2. Non-pharmacologic therapies:
   a. Physiotherapy
   b. Occupational therapy
   c. Education for joint protection and preservation

    d. Orthotics and splints

    e. Heat and cold therapy

    f. Hydrotherapy

    g. Adaptive equipment

3. Pharmacologic therapy:

    a. Non-biologic DMARDS are first-line treatment options:

    Methotrexate, Cyclosporine, Sulphasalazine, Leflunomide, Ustekinumab (Anti IL 12/23)

    b. TNF alpha inhibitors: Certolizumab pegol

    c. Newer drugs: Apremilast (Inhibitor of Phosphodiesterase 4)

    d. Treatment of psoriasis

    e. Others: NSAIDs, Corticosteroids, other analgesics

4. Surgical treatments: Synovectomy, arthrodesis and reconstructive surgery or arthroplasty.

Case No 3: Polymyositis/ Dermatomyositis

Aetiology

Polymyositis: Idiopathic inflammatory myositis with symmetrical proximal myopathy, elevated creatinine kinase levels, and characteristic myopathic changes on electromyography.

Dermatomyositis: Idiopathic inflammatory myositis with cutaneous manifestations and proximal myopathy.

Management

Investigations

Blood Tests

1. Full blood count
2. Urea and electrolytes
3. Liver function tests
4. Erythrocyte sedimentation rate
5. Rheumatoid factor assay
6. C-reactive protein
7. Creatinine kinase level
8. Lactate dehydrogenase
9. Anti-nuclear antibody level
10. Myositis-specific antibodies
11. Antisynthetase antibodies: Anti-Jo11

12. Signal recognition peptide antibodies: Increased risk of cardiac involvement and higher mortality.
13. Anti-PM/Scl, anti-Ku - overlapping features of myositis and scleroderma
14. Tumour markers if suspected malignancy

Imaging Studies
1. MRI - best modality to confirm muscle involvement, oedema, inflammation
2. Electromyography
3. Chest X-ray
4. CT if suspected malignancy
5. Mammography/ upper and lower GI endoscopy and pelvic ultrasonography for suspected malignancy

Others
1. Urinalysis for myoglobinuria
2. Muscle biopsy
3. Electrocardiogram
4. Echocardiography
5. Lung function tests
6. Oesophageal manometry

Treatment

General Measures
1. Patient education and advice
2. Promoting a healthy lifestyle - diet/ exercise/ stop smoking
3. Look at other aspects of lifestyle - Cutting down on alcohol intake, advice against recreational drug use

Specific Measures

1. Refer to a rheumatologist and dermatologist
2. Non-pharmacologic therapies:
   a. Physiotherapy
   b. Occupational therapy
   c. Education for joint protection and preservation
   d. Orthotics and splints
   e. Heat and cold therapy
   f. Hydrotherapy
   g. Adaptive equipment
   h. Multi-disciplinary involvement - speech and language therapists, dieticians, social workers, renal, respiratory, gastrointestinal, neurology, oncology and cardiology specialists
3. Pharmacologic therapy:
   a. Corticosteroids
   b. Immunosuppressants:

      Azathioprine, Cyclophosphamide, Chlorambucil,

      Cyclosporine, Methotrexate, Leflunomide, Mycophenolate mofetil
   c. Intravenous immunoglobulin
   d. Sun protection measures
   e. Calcium channel blockers for calcinosis along with bisphosphonates
   f. Treatment of cancer, if appropriate

Case No 4: Systemic Lupus Erythematosus

Aetiology

Systemic lupus erythematosus (SLE) is a chronic systemic autoimmune disease with multi-organ involvement.

The American College of Rheumatology criteria for diagnosis of SLE: The presence of 4 of the 11 criteria indicates good sensitivity and specificity for SLE

- a. Malar rash
- b. Discoid rash
- c. Serositis
- d. Arthritis
- e. Oral ulcers
- f. Renal involvement
- g. Haematological involvement
- h. Neurological involvement
- i. Immunological phenomena - anti dsDNA, anti-Smith antibodies
- j. Photosensitivity
- k. Anti-nuclear antibodies

Management

Investigations

Blood Tests

1. Full blood count
2. Urea and electrolytes
3. Liver function tests
4. Erythrocyte sedimentation rate
5. Rheumatoid factor assay
6. C-reactive protein
7. Creatinine kinase level
8. Lactate dehydrogenase
9. Anti-nuclear antibody level
10. Complement levels - C3 and C4
11. Extractable nuclear antigens:
    Anti-ribonucleoprotein, Anti-Ro/SSA, anti-La/SSB,
    Anti-dsDNA and Anti-Smith antibodies
12. Anticardiolipin, lupus anticoagulant and beta-2
    glycoprotein 1 antibodies

Imaging Studies

1. Chest X-ray
2. Cardiac MRI
3. MRI - to look for vasculitis
4. Joint X-rays

Others Investigations

1. Joint aspiration
2. Muscle, skin and renal biopsy

3. Electrocardiogram
4. Echocardiography
5. Lumbar puncture

Treatment

General Measures

1. Patient education and advice
2. Promoting a healthy lifestyle - diet/ exercise/ stop smoking
3. Look at other aspects of lifestyle - Cutting down on alcohol intake, advice against recreational drug use

Specific Measures

1. Refer to a rheumatologist
2. Non-pharmacologic therapies:
   a. Physiotherapy
   b. Exercise
   c. Occupational therapy
   d. Education for joint protection and preservation
   e. Orthotics and splints
   f. Heat and cold therapy
   g. Hydrotherapy
   h. Adaptive equipment
   i. Multi-disciplinary involvement - speech and language therapists, dieticians, social workers, renal, respiratory, gastrointestinal, haematology, dermatology, neurology and cardiology specialists
3. Pharmacologic therapy:

a. Glucocorticoids, NSAIDS and antimalarial agents for those without major organ involvement

b. Immunosuppressive therapy with Azathioprine, Mycophenolate mofetil and Methotrexate

c. Sun protection

d. Biologic DMARDS: Belimumab (B lymphocyte stimulator specific inhibitor), Rituximab (B cell depletion)

e. Lupus nephritis - managed by the specialist nephrology team - may need renal replacement therapy in the form of dialysis or transplant for end-stage renal failure

f. Prompt obstetrician involvement for pregnant lupus patients

g. Bone protection - Vitamin D (because of sun avoidance)

h. Contraception and family planning advice

Case No 5: Systemic Sclerosis

Aetiology

Systemic sclerosis is a progressive chronic systemic connective tissue disease with multi-organ involvement.

Types of systemic sclerosis

i. Diffuse systemic sclerosis
ii. Limited systemic sclerosis: Calcinosis, Raynaud's phenomenon, oesophageal dysmotility, sclerodactyly, telangiectasia (CREST Syndrome)
iii. Transitory systemic sclerosis
iv. Systemic scleroderma sine scleroderma
v. Malignant scleroderma

Management

Investigations

Blood Tests

1. Full blood count
2. Urea and electrolytes
3. Liver function tests
4. Erythrocyte sedimentation rate
5. Rheumatoid factor assay
6. C-reactive protein

7. Anti-Topoisomerase 1 DNA (Scl 70) - for diffuse systemic sclerosis
8. Anti-centromere - for limited systemic sclerosis
9. Anti-nuclear antibody level
10. Anti-PM/Scl antibodies - for polymyositis/ systemic sclerosis overlap syndrome
11. Anti-mitochondrial antibody

Imaging Studies
1. Chest X-ray
2. High-resolution CT chest
3. Joint X-rays, if appropriate

Other Investigations
1. Oesophageal manometry
2. Skin and renal biopsy
3. Electrocardiogram
4. Echocardiography
5. Lung function tests
6. Broncho alveolar lavage
7. Capillaroscopy

Treatment
General Measures
1. Patient education and advice
2. Promoting a healthy lifestyle - diet/ exercise/ stop smoking
3. Look at other aspects of lifestyle - Cutting down on alcohol intake, advice against recreational drug use

Specific Measures

1. Refer to a rheumatologist
2. Non-pharmacologic therapies:
    a. Physiotherapy
    b. Exercise
    c. Occupational therapy
    d. Education for joint protection and preservation
    e. Orthotics and splints
    f. Heat and cold therapy
    g. Hydrotherapy
    h. Adaptive equipment
    i. Avoiding exposure to cold, gloves
    j. Multi-disciplinary involvement – speech and language therapists, dieticians, social workers, renal, respiratory, gastrointestinal, haematology, dermatology, and cardiology specialists
3. Pharmacological therapy:
    a. Calcium channel blockers, vasodilators, prostaglandin analogues for Raynaud's phenomenon
    b. ACE inhibitors or Angiotensin II receptor antagonists for renal involvement
    c. H2 blockers and proton pump inhibitors for gastrointestinal involvement
    d. Antifibrotic agents- D-penicillamine, interferon alpha and gamma
    e. Other agents: Corticosteroids, Cyclosporine, Methotrexate, Chlorambucil, Cyclophosphamide
4. Surgical management for telangiectasias

Case No 6: Gout

Aetiology

Gout is a crystal arthropathy resulting from the deposition of monosodium urate crystals in the affected joints.

Management

Investigations

Blood Tests

1. Full blood count
2. Urea and electrolytes
3. Liver function tests
4. Erythrocyte sedimentation rate
5. Rheumatoid factor assay
6. C-reactive protein
7. Serum urate level
8. Lipid levels
9. Fasting blood glucose and HbA1C
10. Serum calcium, magnesium, phosphate and iron levels
11. Thyroid function tests

Imaging Studies

1. X-rays of affected joints

2. Ultrasonography of joints
3. CT of affected joints
4. MRI - if tendon sheath involvement and suspicion of osteomyelitis

Other Investigations

1. Joint aspiration and synovial fluid analysis - negatively birefringent urate crystals under polarised light microscopy
2. Urinary uric acid levels

Treatment

General Measures

1. Patient education and advice
2. Promoting a healthy lifestyle - diet/ exercise/ stop smoking
3. Look at other aspects of lifestyle - Cutting down on alcohol intake, advice against recreational drug use

Specific Measures

1. Refer to a rheumatologist
2. Non-pharmacologic therapies:
   a. Physiotherapy
   b. Exercise
   c. Occupational therapy
   d. Education for joint protection and preservation
   e. Orthotics and splints
   f. Heat and cold therapy
   g. Hydrotherapy

    h. Adaptive equipment

    i. Dietician involvement - to avoid purine-rich foods

3. Pharmacological therapy:

    a. Treatment of acute attack: NSAIDs, colchicines or corticosteroids

    b. Treatment of chronic gout:

        i. Xanthine oxidase inhibitors: Allopurinol, Febuxostat

        ii. Rasburicase - for prevention of tumour lysis syndrome in patients undergoing chemotherapy

        iii. Uricosuric agents:

           Probenecid, Benzbromarone

        iv. Others: Synthetic ACTH

Case No 7: Ankylosing Spondylitis

Aetiology

Ankylosing spondylitis is a chronic, inflammatory spondyloarthropathy mainly involving the sacroiliac joints and the axial skeleton but can progress to a multi-system involvement.

Management

Investigations

Blood Tests

1. Full blood count
2. Urea and electrolytes
3. Liver function tests
4. Erythrocyte sedimentation rate
5. Rheumatoid factor assay
6. C-reactive protein
7. Anti-nuclear antibody assay
8. Serum immunoglobulin levels
9. Serum urate level
10. HLA B27 level

Imaging Studies

1. Plain X-ray of the lumbosacral spine – bamboo spine in advanced disease

2. MRI of the entire spine
3. CT of sacroiliac joints

Other Investigations

1. Investigations for extra-articular manifestations as appropriate

Treatment

General Measures

1. Patient education and advice
2. Promoting a healthy lifestyle - diet/ exercise/ stop smoking
3. Look at other aspects of lifestyle - Cutting down on alcohol intake, advice against recreational drug use

Specific Measures

1. Refer to a rheumatologist
2. Non-pharmacologic therapies:
   a. Physiotherapy
   b. Exercise
   c. Occupational therapy
   d. Education for joint protection and preservation
   e. Orthotics and splints
   f. Heat and cold therapy
   g. Hydrotherapy
   h. Adaptive equipment
3. Pharmacological therapy:
   a. NSAIDs and corticosteroids

b. DMARDS:

Sulphasalazine, Methotrexate, Azathioprine, Cyclophosphamide and Cyclosporine

c. TNF-alpha inhibitors: Etanercept, Infliximab, Adalimumab, Golimumab, Certolizumab pegol

d. Treatment of extra-articular manifestations as appropriate

4. Surgical management: Joint replacement, vertebral osteotomy

Case No 8: Osteoarthritis

Aetiology

Osteoarthritis is the most common degenerative arthritis with no particular systemic involvement.

Management

Investigations

Blood Tests

1. Full blood count
2. Urea and electrolytes
3. Liver function tests
4. Erythrocyte sedimentation rate
5. Rheumatoid factor assay
6. C-reactive protein
7. Anti-nuclear antibody assay
8. Serum urate level
9. Lipid levels

Imaging Studies

1. Plain X-ray of affected joints
2. CT of affected joints
3. Bone scan
4. MRI and ultrasonography if additional pathology suspected

Other Investigations

1. Joint aspiration

Treatment

General Measures

1. Patient education and advice
2. Promoting a healthy lifestyle - diet/ exercise/ stop smoking
3. Look at other aspects of lifestyle - Cutting down on alcohol intake, advice against recreational drug use

Specific Measures

1. Refer to a rheumatologist
2. Non-pharmacologic therapies:
    a. Physiotherapy
    b. Exercise
    c. Occupational therapy
    d. Weight loss
    e. Heat and cold therapy
    f. Hydrotherapy
    g. Adaptive equipment
3. Pharmacological therapy:
    a. NSAIDs - oral and topical
    b. Other analgesics
4. Surgical management: Osteotomy, arthroscopy, joint replacement, fusion

Case No 9: Proximal Myopathy

Aetiology

Multiple: Idiopathic, inflammatory, infectious, metabolic, drug-induced, endocrine or congenital

Management

Investigations

Blood Tests

1. Full blood count
2. Urea and electrolytes
3. Liver function tests
4. Erythrocyte sedimentation rate
5. Rheumatoid factor assay
6. C-reactive protein
7. Serum myoglobulin level
8. Extractable nuclear antigen level
9. Anti-nuclear antibody level
10. Lipid levels
11. Anti mitochondrial antibody
12. Thyroid function tests
13. Anti-histone antibodies
14. Creatinine kinase levels
15. Serum calcium, magnesium, phosphate, and iron levels
16. Genetic testing

Imaging Studies

1. MRI

Other Investigations

1. Muscle biopsy
2. Electromyography
3. Electrocardiogram
4. Echocardiography

Treatment

General measures

1. Patient education and advice
2. Promoting a healthy lifestyle - diet/ exercise/ stop smoking
3. Look at other aspects of lifestyle - Cutting down on alcohol intake, advice against recreational drug use

Specific Measures

1. Refer to a rheumatologist
2. Non-pharmacologic therapies:
   a. Physiotherapy
   b. Exercise
   c. Occupational therapy
   d. Adaptive equipment
3. Pharmacological therapy:
   a. Treatment of any underlying cause

Case No 10: Rarer Cases

A] Charcot Arthropathy

Points to remember

1. Neuropathic joint - progressive destruction leading to deformities
2. Seen commonly as a complication of diabetes
3. Other causes for Charcot joint - leprosy, syphilis, syringomyelia, patients with end-stage renal failure on dialysis, chronic alcoholism
4. Management is mainly conservative with rest and immobilisation in total contact casts in the acute phase.
5. Surgical management in the form of osteotomy, arthrodesis, reconstructive surgery and internal fixation may also be considered

B] Paget's Disease

Points to remember

1. Disorder of bone remodelling, which involves excessive bone resorption followed by increased bone formation
2. Familial Paget's disease - associated with mutations in SQSTM1/p62
3. Important blood tests include serum alkaline phosphatase, bone-specific alkaline phosphatase,

urinary hydroxyproline, along with serum calcium, phosphate and parathyroid hormone levels
4. Plain X-rays and Bone scans are the best imaging modalities, along with CT and MRI when indicated.
5. Bisphosphonates and calcitonin remain the mainstay of treatment

C] Vasculitis

Points to remember

1. Inflammation of the blood vessels leading to multi-organ involvement
2. Classification:
   a. Large vessel vasculitis: Takayasu's arteritis
   b. Medium vessel vasculitis: Kawasaki disease, polyarteritis nodosa
   c. Small vessel vasculitis: Microscopic polyangiitis, Wegener's granulomatosis, Churg Strauss Syndrome, Henoch-Schoenlein purpura, leukocytoclastic vasculitis
   d. Others: Behcet's disease, anti-GBM syndrome
3. A rheumatological screen must be performed in patients suspected of having a vasculitis, with specific antibodies in the event of recognition of a type of vasculitides.
4. Vascular imaging in the form of angiography is considered helpful
5. Treatment involves an induction phase with high-dose corticosteroids and Cyclophosphamide, with Rituximab gaining some evidence for use in this phase. Maintenance phase with either Cyclophosphamide or Rituximab has been used, with Methotrexate and Azathioprine as alternatives.

D] Jaccoud's Arthropathy

Points to remember

1. Deforming non-erosive arthropathy
2. Associated with several rheumatic and non-rheumatic conditions such as systemic lupus erythematosus, connective tissue diseases, psoriatic arthritis and inflammatory bowel disease
3. Investigations and management depend on the cause

E] Marfan Syndrome

Points to remember

1. Autosomal dominant connective tissue disease
2. Defect in FBN1 gene on chromosome 15, which codes for fibrillin
3. Monitoring the cardiovascular system is of utmost importance given the cardiac involvement, with regular echocardiograms and measurement of aortic root diameter
4. Slit lamp examination for lens abnormalities and keratometry is advised
5. Symptomatic management with prompt treatment of cardiac complications is of utmost importance.

F] Mixed Connective Tissue Disease

Points to remember

1. Overlap syndrome commonly occurs with systemic lupus erythematosus, scleroderma and myositis
2. Anti U1 Ribonucleoprotein and anti U1 - 70kd are present

3. A complete rheumatological screen must be performed
4. Treatment depends on the primary disease and the symptoms

Brief Clinical Consultations: Dermatology

Case No 1: Psoriasis

Aetiology

Psoriasis is a chronic, inflammatory disease mainly involving hyperproliferation of keratinocytes in the epidermis. As a result, there is an increase in epidermal cell turnover.

Management

Investigations

Blood Tests

1. Full blood count
2. Urea and electrolytes
3. Liver function tests
4. Erythrocyte sedimentation rate
5. Hepatitis panel
6. C-reactive protein
7. Rheumatoid factor level
8. Serum urate level

Imaging Studies

1. Plain X-rays of any affected joints
2. Bone scans when appropriate

Other Investigations

1. Skin biopsy
2. Auspitz sign – the appearance of punctate bleeding spots when psoriatic scales are scraped off

Treatment

General Measures

1. Patient education and advice
2. Promoting a healthy lifestyle - diet/ exercise/ stop smoking
3. Look at other aspects of lifestyle - Cutting down on alcohol intake, advice against recreational drug use

Specific Measures

1. Refer to a dermatologist
2. Stress reduction
3. Light therapy - psoralen UVA/ narrowband UVB
4. Medications:
   Corticosteroids, Coal tar, Anthralin, Vitamin D analogues, Topical retinoids, Methotrexate, Tacrolimus, Cyclosporine, Ustekinumab, TNF-alpha inhibitors - Infliximab, Etanercept, Adalimumab
5. Refer to an ophthalmologist for ocular complications

Case No 2: Eczema

Aetiology

Unknown aetiology causing a pruritic disease

Management

Investigations

Blood Tests

1. Full blood count
2. Urea and electrolytes
3. Liver function tests
4. Erythrocyte sedimentation rate
5. Hepatitis panel
6. C-reactive protein
7. Rheumatoid factor level
8. Serum urate level

Imaging Studies

1. Plain X-rays of any affected joints
2. Bone scans when appropriate

Other Investigations

1. Skin biopsy
2. Swab from an infected area if there is one or more

3. Allergy and radioallergosorbent testing (RAST)
4. Skin scraping

Treatment

General Measures

1. Patient education and advice
2. Promoting a healthy lifestyle - diet/ exercise/ stop smoking
3. Look at other aspects of lifestyle - Cutting down on alcohol intake, advice against recreational drug use

Specific Measures

1. Refer to a dermatologist
2. Topical steroids
3. Emollients and moisturisers
4. Immunomodulators - Tacrolimus, Pimecrolimus, Omalizumab
5. Phototherapy
6. Antibiotics for infections
7. Treatment of allergies
8. Dietician review and advice

Case No 3: Dermatomyositis

Aetiology

Dermatomyositis is an idiopathic inflammatory myositis with cutaneous manifestations and proximal myopathy.

Management

Investigations

Blood Tests

1. Full blood count
2. Urea and electrolytes
3. Liver function tests
4. Erythrocyte sedimentation rate
5. Rheumatoid factor assay
6. C-reactive protein
7. Creatinine kinase level
8. Lactate dehydrogenase
9. Anti-nuclear antibody level
10. Myositis-specific antibodies
11. Antisynthetase antibodies: Anti-Jo-1
12. Signal recognition peptide antibodies: Increased risk of cardiac involvement and higher mortality
13. Anti-PM/Scl, anti-Ku - overlapping features of myositis and scleroderma
14. Tumour markers if suspected malignancy

Imaging Studies

1. MRI - the best modality to confirm muscle involvement, oedema, inflammation
2. Electromyography
3. Chest X-ray
4. CT if suspected malignancy
5. Mammography/ upper and lower GI endoscopy and pelvic ultrasonography for suspected malignancy

Other Investigations

1. Urinalysis for myoglobinuria
2. Muscle biopsy
3. Electrocardiogram
4. Echocardiography
5. Lung function tests
6. Oesophageal manometry

Treatment

General Measures

1. Patient education and advice
2. Promoting a healthy lifestyle - diet/ exercise/ stop smoking
3. Look at other aspects of lifestyle - Cutting down on alcohol intake, advice against recreational drug use

Specific Measures

1. Refer to a rheumatologist and dermatologist
2. Non-pharmacologic therapies:
   a. Physiotherapy

b. Occupational therapy

c. Education for joint protection and preservation

d. Orthotics and splints

e. Heat and cold therapy

f. Hydrotherapy

g. Adaptive equipment

h. Multi-disciplinary involvement - speech and language therapists, dieticians, social workers, renal, respiratory, gastrointestinal, oncology, neurology and cardiology specialists

3. Pharmacologic therapy:

a. Corticosteroids

b. Immunosuppressants:

Azathioprine, Cyclophosphamide, Chlorambucil, Cyclosporine, Methotrexate, Leflunomide, Mycophenolate mofetil

c. Intravenous Immunoglobulin

d. Sun protection measures

e. Calcium channel blockers for calcinosis along with bisphosphonates

f. Treatment of cancer, if appropriate

Case No 4: Tuberous Sclerosis

Aetiology

Tuberous Sclerosis is an autosomal dominant disorder with multi-organ involvement - mainly renal, cutaneous and neurological.

Important points to remember

a. Neurological findings: Subependymal nodules
b. Dermatological findings: Adenoma sebaceum, ash leaf macules, periungual and gingival fibromas, and shagreen patch.
c. Cardiac findings: Rhabdomyomas
d. Ophthalmological findings: Retinal astrocytomas
e. Pulmonary findings: Lung cysts, lymphangiomyomatosis
f. Renal findings: Polycystic kidney disease, renal cysts, angiomyolipoma, renal cell carcinoma

Management

Investigations

Blood Tests

1. Full blood count
2. Urea and electrolytes
3. Liver function tests

4. Erythrocyte sedimentation rate
5. Rheumatoid factor assay
6. C-reactive protein
7. Genetic testing

Imaging Studies
1. CT of the brain/ chest/ abdomen and pelvis
2. MRI brain
3. Renal ultrasound

Other Investigations
1. Electrocardiogram
2. Echocardiogram
3. Electroencephalogram

Treatment

General Measures
1. Patient education and advice
2. Promoting a healthy lifestyle - diet/ exercise/ stop smoking
3. Look at other aspects of lifestyle - Cutting down on alcohol intake, advice against recreational drug use

Specific Measures
1. Refer to all the necessary specialities as mentioned with multi-organ involvement
2. mTOR kinase inhibitors - Everolimus
3. Treatment of complications - anti-epileptics, benzodiazepines, corticosteroids

Case No 5: Systemic Sclerosis

Aetiology

Systemic sclerosis is a progressive chronic systemic connective tissue disease with multi-organ involvement.

Types of systemic sclerosis

i.   Diffuse systemic sclerosis
ii. Limited Systemic sclerosis: Calcinosis, Raynaud's phenomenon, oesophageal dysmotility, sclerodactyly, telangiectasia (CREST Syndrome)
iii. Transitory systemic sclerosis
iv. Systemic scleroderma sine scleroderma
v.   Malignant scleroderma

Management

Investigations

Blood Tests

1. Full blood count
2. Urea and electrolytes
3. Liver function tests
4. Erythrocyte sedimentation rate
5. Rheumatoid factor assay
6. C-reactive protein

7. Anti-Topoisomerase 1 (anti-Scl-70) - for diffuse systemic sclerosis

8. Anti-centromere - for limited systemic sclerosis

9. Anti-nuclear antibody level

10. Anti-PM/Scl antibodies - for polymyositis/ systemic sclerosis overlap syndrome

11. Anti-mitochondrial antibody

Imaging Studies

1. Chest X-ray

2. High-resolution CT chest

3. Joint X-rays, if appropriate

Other Investigations

1. Oesophageal manometry

2. Skin and renal biopsy

3. Electrocardiogram

4. Echocardiography

5. Lung function tests

6. Broncho alveolar lavage

7. Capillaroscopy

Treatment

General Measures

1. Patient education and advice

2. Promoting a healthy lifestyle - diet/ exercise/ stop smoking

3. Look at other aspects of lifestyle - Cutting down on alcohol intake, advice against recreational drug use

Specific Measures

1. Refer to a rheumatologist
2. Non-pharmacologic therapies:
    a. Physiotherapy
    b. Exercise
    c. Occupational therapy
    d. Education for joint protection and preservation
    e. Orthotics and splints
    f. Heat and cold therapy
    g. Hydrotherapy
    h. Adaptive equipment
    i. Avoiding exposure to cold, gloves
    j. Multi-disciplinary involvement - speech and language therapists, dieticians, social workers, renal, respiratory, gastrointestinal, haematology, dermatology, and cardiology specialists
3. Pharmacological therapy:
    a. Calcium channel blockers, vasodilators, prostaglandin analogues for Raynaud's phenomenon
    b. ACE inhibitors or angiotensin II receptor antagonists for renal involvement
    c. H2 blockers and proton pump inhibitors for gastrointestinal involvement
    d. Antifibrotic agents - D-penicillamine, interferon-alpha and gamma
    e. Other agents: Corticosteroids, Cyclosporine, Methotrexate, Chlorambucil, Cyclophosphamide
4. Surgical management for telangiectasias

Case No 6: Neurofibromatosis

Aetiology

Autosomal dominant disorder

Types

Neurofibromatosis type I: Central Neurofibromatosis: NF1 gene localised to Chromosome 17

Neurofibromatosis type II: Mutation in chromosome 22

Clinical criteria for the diagnosis of Neurofibromatosis I: Requires 2 out 7 criteria for diagnosis:

    a. 6 or more cafe au lait spots are more than 5mm in diameter in younger than 10 years and 15mm in adults

    b. Axillary or inguinal freckling

    c. Optic nerve glioma

    d. 2 or more neurofibromas or one plexiform neurofibroma

    e. 2 or more iris hamartomas (Lisch nodules)

    f. Sphenoid dysplasia

    g. First-degree relative with neurofibromatosis type I

Management

Investigations

Blood Tests

1. Full blood count
2. Urea and electrolytes
3. Liver function tests
4. Erythrocyte sedimentation rate
5. Rheumatoid factor assay
6. C-reactive protein
7. Genetic testing
8. Plasma catecholamines

Imaging Studies

1. Plain X-rays of affected bones
2. CT brain
3. MRI brain
4. PET scanning

Other Investigations

1. Electrocardiogram
2. Echocardiogram
3. Electroencephalogram
4. Biopsy of neurofibroma
5. Slit lamp examination
6. Urinary catecholamines

Treatment

General Measures

1. Patient education and advice
2. Promoting a healthy lifestyle - diet/ exercise/ stop smoking
3. Look at other aspects of lifestyle - Cutting down on alcohol intake, advice against recreational drug use

Specific Measures

1. Refer to a dermatologist, neurologist, neurosurgeon, ophthalmologist and other specialists as appropriate
2. Surgical removal of neurofibromas, if appropriate
3. Treatment of complications
4. Chemotherapy and radiotherapy for malignancy peripheral nerve sheath tumours and benign intradural extramedullary spinal cord tumours

Case No 7: Vitiligo

Aetiology

An acquired pigmentary disorder characterised by well-circumscribed depigmented macules and patches.

Management

Investigations

Blood Tests

1. Full blood count
2. Urea and electrolytes
3. Liver function tests
4. Erythrocyte sedimentation rate
5. Autoimmune screen
6. Antinuclear antibody
7. Serum antithyroglobulin
8. Serum antithyroid peroxidase
9. Fasting glucose and HbA1

Other Investigations

1. Skin biopsy

Treatment

General Measures

1. Patient education and advice
2. Promoting a healthy lifestyle - diet/ exercise/ stop smoking
3. Look at other aspects of lifestyle - Cutting down on alcohol intake, advice against recreational drug use

Specific Measures

1. Refer to dermatologist
2. Systemic phototherapy
3. Systemic corticosteroids
4. Topical therapy - tacrolimus, vitamin D analogues
5. Sunscreen and skin protection

Case No 8: Raynaud's Phenomenon

Aetiology

Vasospasm leading to discolouration and discomfort affecting mainly fingers and toes in affected individuals

Types

a. Primary Raynaud's phenomenon or Raynaud's disease: Not associated with other diseases

b. Secondary Raynaud's phenomenon: Secondary to other diseases, most commonly autoimmune diseases

Management

Investigations

Blood Tests

1. Full blood count
2. Urea and electrolytes
3. Liver function tests
4. Erythrocyte sedimentation rate
5. Autoimmune screen
6. Antinuclear antibody
7. Thyroid function tests
8. Cold agglutinins
9. Fasting glucose and HbA1

10. Serum viscosity
11. Serum metanephrines and catecholamines
12. Serum protein electrophoresis
13. Antiphospholipid antibody levels
14. Serum creatinine kinase
15. Serum leucocyte alkaline phosphatase
16. Growth hormone levels
17. Heavy metal screen
18. Clotting studies

Imaging Studies

1. Arteriography
2. Doppler ultrasound

Other Investigations

1. Nail fold capillaroscopy
2. Digital artery pressure

Treatment

General Measures

1. Patient education and advice
2. Promoting a healthy lifestyle - diet/ exercise/ stop smoking
3. Look at other aspects of lifestyle - Cutting down on alcohol intake, advice against recreational drug use

Specific Measures

1. Refer to a dermatologist, rheumatologist
2. Hand warming - gloves

3. Calcium channel blockers - Nifedipine
4. Angiotensin receptor blockers and prostaglandin analogues
5. Avoidance of trigger
6. Topical nitro-glycerine
7. Treatment of any underlying disorder

Case No 9: Henoch-Schönlein Purpura

Aetiology

IgA medicated small vessel vasculitis with multi-organ involvement.

Management

Investigations

Blood Tests

1. Full blood count
2. Urea and electrolytes
3. Liver function tests
4. Erythrocyte sedimentation rate
5. Amylase and lipase
6. Antinuclear antibody
7. Clotting studies
8. D-dimer
9. Fasting glucose and HbA1
10. Serum viscosity
11. Rheumatoid factor
12. Serum IgA level
13. CH50 level
14. Complement levels – C3 and C4

Imaging Studies

1. Abdominal ultrasound
2. CT brain
3. MRI brain

Other Investigations

1. Urinalysis
2. Renal biopsy
3. Endoscopy

Treatment

General Measures

1. Patient education and advice
2. Promoting a healthy lifestyle - diet/ exercise/ stop smoking
3. Look at other aspects of lifestyle - Cutting down on alcohol intake, advice against recreational drug use

Specific Measures

1. Refer to a dermatologist, rheumatologist, renal physician
2. Supportive management - IV fluids, analgesics
3. Induction treatment with corticosteroids and Cyclophosphamide
4. Other treatments: Azathioprine, Cyclosporine, Dipyridamole, Intravenous Immunoglobulin G
5. Plasmapheresis

Case No 10: Rarer Cases

A] Urticaria

Points to remember

1. Pruritic well-circumscribed lesions associated with erythema and oedema
2. Always ask for precipitants
3. Antihistamines and H2 receptor blockers are used in the management
4. Tricyclic antidepressants and corticosteroids are also used in the management

B] Osler-Weber-Rendu Syndrome

Points to remember

1. Also known as hereditary haemorrhagic telangiectasia (HHT)
2. An autosomal dominant disorder affecting blood vessels leading to telangiectasias and bleeding
3. Characterised by mucocutaneous and arteriovenous malformations.
4. Recurrent epistaxis, GI bleeding and pulmonary haemorrhage are important complications to be considered

C] Gouty Tophi

Points to remember

1. Re-visit the topic of gout as described in the rheumatology section
2. Composition - monosodium urate crystals
3. Crystals exhibit negative birefringence in polarised light
4. Investigations and management as above

D] Ehler Danlos Syndrome

Points to remember

1. Autosomal dominant connective tissue disease resulting from a genetic defect in collagen
2. Hypermobility is confirmed by using the Beighton scoring system: A score of 5 or more confirms hypermobility:
   a. One point for passive dorsiflexion of each fifth finger >90°
   b. One point for passive apposition of each thumb to the flexor surface of the forearm
   c. One point for hyperextension of each elbow >10°
   d. One point for hyperextension of each knee >10°
   e. One point for the ability to place the palms on the floor with the knees fully extended
3. The Brighton criteria are used to diagnose Hypermobility syndrome: 2 major/ 1 major + 2 minor/ 4 minor criteria:
   a. Major criteria

- A Beighton score of 4/9 or more (either current or historic)
- Arthralgia for more than three months in four or more joints

b. Minor criteria
- A Beighton score of 1, 2 or 3/9 (0, 1, 2 or 3 if aged 50+)
- Arthralgia (> 3 months) in one to three joints or back pain (> 3 months), spondylosis, spondylolysis/spondylolisthesis
- Dislocation/subluxation in more than one joint or one joint on more than one occasion
- Soft tissue rheumatism. > 3 lesions (e.g. epicondylitis, tenosynovitis, bursitis).
- Marfanoid habitus (tall, slim, span/height ratio >1.03, upper: lower segment ratio less than 0.89, arachnodactyly (positive Steinberg thumb / Walker wrist signs)
- Abnormal skin: striae, hyperextensibility, thin skin, papyraceous scarring
- Eye signs: drooping eyelids, myopia or antimongoloid slant (Palpebral slant)
- Varicose veins or hernia or uterine/rectal prolapse

E] Pseudoxanthoma Elasticum

Points to remember

1. Autosomal recessive disease with a mutation in the ABCC6 gene in the short arm of chromosome 16
2. Cutaneous manifestations include skin laxity,

yellow papules and plaques, plucked chicken appearance

3. Extra cutaneous manifestations include angioid retinal streaks, mitral valve prolapse, GI haemorrhage, hypertension, and rarely cerebrovascular accident and haematuria

F] Diabetic Dermopathy/ Necrobiosis Lipoidica Diabeticorum

Points to remember

1. Disorder of collagen degeneration with a granulomatous response, blood vessel abnormalities and fat deposition
2. Most commonly seen over the pretibial area
3. Also seen in patients with rheumatoid arthritis

G] Skin Malignancy

Points to remember

Basal Cell Carcinoma

1. Most common skin cancer which rarely metastasises
2. Common types: Superficial/ infiltrative/ nodular
3. Most commonly noted over the face/ head/ arms
4. Often has a pearly appearance with a central ulceration
5. Surgery is the mainstay of treatment
6. Chemotherapy, radiotherapy, and photodynamic therapy are other modes of treatment

Squamous Cell Carcinoma

1. Second most common skin cancer, affecting the head and neck regions
2. Presents as a shallow ulcer with heaped edges, usually in sun-exposed areas
3. Surgery remains the mainstay of treatment
4. Mohs microdissection surgery, electro-dissection and curettage, radiotherapy and chemotherapy are other options

Malignant Melanoma

1. To differentiate melanoma from benign naevus:
   a. A: Asymmetry
   b. B: Border irregularity
   c. C: Colour variation
   d. D: Diameter > 6mm
   e. E: Enlarging or evolving
2. Histologic types of melanomas:
   a. Superficial spreading melanoma
   b. Nodular melanoma
   c. Lentigo maligna melanoma
   d. Acral lentiginous melanoma
   e. Mucosal lentiginous melanoma
   f. Amelanotic melanoma
3. Clark's level and Breslow's depth are used for staging purposes
4. BRAF mutations are present in 40 - 60% of melanomas
5. Initial treatment for early melanomas involves surgery

6. Adjuvant chemotherapy is offered to high-risk patients

7. Dacarbazine was one of the initial few drugs approved for the treatment of advanced melanoma

8. Other drugs: Carboplatin, Paclitaxel, Ipilimumab, and the BRAF inhibitors - Vemurafenib

9. Prevention is better than cure - Avoidance of sun exposure in at-risk individuals

Brief Clinical Consultations: Endocrinology

Case No 1: Acromegaly

Aetiology

Acromegaly is due to excessive growth hormone production leading to characteristic features of gigantism and multi-organ involvement.

Management

Investigations

Blood Tests

1. Full blood count
2. Urea and electrolytes
3. Liver function tests
4. Growth hormone level
5. Serum insulin-like growth factor 1 level
6. Growth hormone-releasing hormone levels
7. Prolactin level
8. Fasting glucose and HbA1

Imaging Studies

1. CT brain
2. MRI brain

Treatment

General Measures

1. Patient education and advice
2. Promoting a healthy lifestyle - diet/ exercise/ stop smoking
3. Look at other aspects of lifestyle - Cutting down on alcohol intake, advice against recreational drug use

Specific Measures

1. Refer to an Endocrinologist
2. Pharmacological therapy:
   a. Somatostatin analogues - Octreotide, Lanreotide
   b. Dopamine receptor agonists - Bromocriptine, Cabergoline
   c. Growth hormone receptor antagonists - Pegvisomant
3. Other treatment options:
   a. Radiotherapy
   b. Trans-sphenoidal resection

Case No 2: Graves' Disease

Aetiology

An autoimmune disease, leading mainly to hyperthyroidism and its associated manifestations.

Management

Investigations

Blood Tests

1. Full blood count
2. Urea and electrolytes
3. Liver function tests
4. Thyroid function tests
5. Thyrotropin-releasing hormone
6. Fasting lipids
7. Serum testosterone level
8. Fasting glucose and HbA1

Imaging Studies

1. Radioactive iodine scan
2. Ultrasound thyroid
3. CT or MRI orbits

Treatment

General Measures

1. Patient education and advice
2. Promoting a healthy lifestyle - diet/ exercise/ stop smoking
3. Look at other aspects of lifestyle - Cutting down on alcohol intake, advice against recreational drug use

Specific Measures

1. Refer to an endocrinologist
2. Pharmacological therapy:
   a. Radioactive iodine
   b. Corticosteroids
   c. Antithyroid drugs: Propylthio uracil, Carbimazole, Methimazole
   d. Beta-blockers: Propranolol, Atenolol
3. Other treatment options:
   a. Orbital radiotherapy
   b. Orbital decompression
   c. Thyroidectomy - not used as the first choice

Case No 3: Hyperthyroidism/ Hypothyroidism

Aetiology

Hyperthyroidism

1. Graves' disease
2. Toxic multinodular goitre
3. Toxic thyroid adenoma
4. Others: Inflammatory - Hashimoto's/ De Quervain's thyroiditis, postpartum thyroiditis, medications - amiodarone

Hypothyroidism

1. Iodine deficiency
2. Previous thyroidectomy
3. Autoimmune thyroiditis
4. Previous radioactive iodine treatment
5. Congenital causes – Pendred syndrome, thyroid dyshormonogenesis
6. Pituitary compression

Management

Investigations

Blood Tests

1. Full blood count
2. Urea and electrolytes
3. Liver function tests
4. Thyroid function tests
5. Thyrotropin-releasing hormone
6. TSH Receptor antibodies
7. Fasting lipids
8. Serum testosterone level
9. Fasting glucose and HbA1
10. Serum Creatinine kinase level

Imaging Studies

1. Thyroid scintigraphy
2. Ultrasound thyroid

Others Investigations

1. Fine Needle Aspiration Biopsy

Treatment

General Measures

1. Patient education and advice
2. Promoting a healthy lifestyle - diet/ exercise/ stop smoking
3. Look at other aspects of lifestyle - Cutting down on alcohol intake, advice against recreational drug use

Specific Measures

1. Refer to an endocrinologist
2. Pharmacological therapy:
   a. Management of ophthalmopathy
   b. Management of dermopathy
   c. Antithyroid drugs: Propylthiouracil, Carbimazole, Methimazole
   d. Radioactive Iodine
   e. Thyroxine replacement for hypothyroidism

Case No 4: Cushing's Syndrome

Aetiology

Excessive exposure to inappropriately high cortisol levels leading to characteristic manifestations

Causes

1. Exogenous administration of glucocorticoids
2. Pituitary adenoma - Cushing's disease
3. Adrenal hyperplasia
4. Adrenocorticotropic hormone (ACTH) producing tumours
5. Corticotrophin-releasing hormone (CRH) secreting tumours

Management

Investigations

Blood Tests

1. Full blood count
2. Urea and electrolytes
3. Liver function tests
4. Serum and urinary cortisol levels
5. Low dose dexamethasone suppression test
6. ACTH level

7. Fasting lipids
8. Fasting glucose and HbA1
9. Autoimmune screen
10. Tumour markers, if indicated

Imaging Studies
1. MRI brain
2. CT abdomen
3. Octreotide scintigraphy
4. CT chest/ abdomen/ pelvis - if malignancy suspected

Other Investigations
1. Urinary-free cortisol - usually the first investigation of choice
2. Inferior petrosal sinus sampling

Treatment

General Measures
1. Patient education and advice
2. Promoting a healthy lifestyle - diet/ exercise/ stop smoking
3. Look at other aspects of lifestyle - Cutting down on alcohol intake, advice against recreational drug use

Specific Measures
1. Refer to an endocrinologist
2. Pharmacological therapy:
   a. Gradual withdrawal of glucocorticoid

   b. Adrenal steroid inhibitors: Metyrapone, Ketoconazole

   c. Glucocorticoid type 2 receptor antagonist: Mifepristone

   d. Somatostatin analogues: Pasireotide - mainly for Cushing's disease

3. Other treatment options:

   a. Abdominal surgery - for adrenalectomy

   b. Transsphenoidal surgery for Cushing's disease

   c. Treatment of malignancy as appropriate

Case No 5: Addison's Disease

Aetiology

A chronic endocrine disorder associated with adrenal insufficiency

Causes

1. Autoimmune adrenalitis
2. Congenital adrenal hypoplasia
3. Chronic granulomatous diseases - Tuberculosis, sarcoidosis, etc
4. Metastatic malignancies
5. Infiltrative disorders - Amyloidosis
6. Acquired immunodeficiency syndrome (AIDS)
7. Medications - Ketoconazole, Busulphan, Etomidate, etc
8. Bilateral adrenal haemorrhage
9. Stress

Management

Investigations

Blood Tests

1. Full blood count
2. Urea and electrolytes

3. Liver function tests
4. ACTH level
5. Fasting lipids
6. Fasting glucose and HbA1
7. Autoimmune screen
8. Tumour markers, if indicated
9. Short synacthen test
10. Serum cortisol level
11. Thyroid function tests
12. Prolactin level

Imaging Studies

1. Chest X-ray
2. CT abdomen

Other Investigations

1. Urinary and sweat sodium
2. Electrocardiogram
3. Sputum examination

Treatment

General Measures

1. Patient education and advice
2. Promoting a healthy lifestyle - diet/ exercise/ stop smoking
3. Look at other aspects of lifestyle - Cutting down on alcohol intake, advice against recreational drug use

Specific Measures

1. Refer to an endocrinologist
2. Pharmacological therapy:
   a. Corticosteroid therapy:
   Prednisolone, Fludrocortisone, Hydrocortisone

Case No 6: Klinefelter Syndrome

Aetiology

Chromosomal disorder with a karyotype of 47 XXY

Management

Investigations

Blood Tests

1. Full blood count
2. Urea and electrolytes
3. Liver function tests
4. Follicular stimulating hormone (FSH) level
5. Luteinising hormone(LH) level
6. Serum testosterone level
7. Oestradiol level
8. Prolactin level
9. Insulin-like growth factor 1 level
10. Cytogenetic studies
11. Clotting studies

Imaging Studies

1. Bone scan
2. Echocardiography

Other Investigations

1. Testicular or breast biopsy

Treatment

General Measures

1. Patient education and advice
2. Promoting a healthy lifestyle - diet/ exercise/ stop smoking
3. Look at other aspects of lifestyle - Cutting down on alcohol intake, advice against recreational drug use

Specific Measures

1. Refer to an endocrinologist
2. Androgen therapy
3. Treatment of infertility
4. Genetic counselling

Case No 7: Turner Syndrome

Aetiology

Chromosomal disorder with the karyotype 45X

Management

Investigations

Blood Tests

1. Full blood count
2. Urea and electrolytes
3. Liver function tests
4. Follicular stimulating hormone level
5. Luteinising hormone level
6. Serum testosterone level
7. Oestradiol level
8. Prolactin level
9. Thyroid function tests
10. Cytogenetic studies
11. Clotting studies
12. Fasting glucose and HbA1C

Imaging Studies

1. Bone scan
2. Echocardiography
3. Renal ultrasound

Other Investigations

1. Audiology

Treatment

General Measures

1. Patient education and advice
2. Promoting a healthy lifestyle - diet/ exercise/ stop smoking
3. Look at other aspects of lifestyle - Cutting down on alcohol intake, advice against recreational drug use

Specific Measures

1. Refer to an endocrinologist, cardiologist and renal physician
2. Oestrogen replacement therapy
3. Growth hormone therapy
4. Genetic counselling

Case No 8: Hypopituitarism

Aetiology

A syndrome due to the deficiency of pituitary hormones

Management

Investigations

Blood Tests

1. Full blood count
2. Urea and electrolytes
3. Liver function tests
4. Follicular stimulating hormone level
5. Luteinising hormone level
6. Serum testosterone level
7. Oestradiol level
8. Prolactin level
9. Thyroid function tests
10. Cytogenetic studies
11. Clotting studies
12. Fasting glucose and HbA1C
13. Serum cortisol level
14. ACTH level
15. Growth hormone level
16. Water Deprivation test
17. Vasopressin stimulation test

Imaging Studies

1. MRI brain

Treatment

General Measures

1. Patient education and advice
2. Promoting a healthy lifestyle - diet/ exercise/ stop smoking
3. Look at other aspects of lifestyle - Cutting down on alcohol intake, advice against recreational drug use

Specific Measures

1. Refer to an endocrinologist
2. Corticosteroids
3. Growth hormone therapy
4. Thyroid hormone replacement
5. Anti-diuretic hormone replacement
6. Oestrogen and progestin therapy
7. Androgen replacement therapy
8. Surgical decompression in cases of pituitary apoplexy

Case No 9: Pseudohypoparathyroidism

Aetiology

Disorder of raised parathyroid hormone levels causing hypocalcaemia and hyperphosphatemia

Management

Investigations

Blood Tests

1. Full blood count
2. Urea and electrolytes
3. Liver function tests
4. Serum calcium level
5. Serum phosphate level
6. Serum parathyroid hormone (PTH) level

Imaging Studies

1. X-rays of the hands
2. CT brain
3. Bone scan

Other Investigations

1. Electrocardiogram

Treatment

General Measures

1. Patient education and advice
2. Promoting a healthy lifestyle - diet/ exercise/ stop smoking
3. Look at other aspects of lifestyle - Cutting down on alcohol intake, advice against recreational drug use

Specific Measures

1. Refer to an endocrinologist
2. Calcium and vitamin D replacement

Case No 10: Other cases

A] Diabetes

Points to remember

1. It's the complications of diabetes that are important for this exam
2. It's important to remember the details of retinopathy, nephropathy and neuropathy
3. Also, remember the macrovascular complications - Cardiovascular disease
4. The different classes of hypoglycaemic agents:
   a. Biguanides: Metformin
   b. Sulphonylureas: Gliclazide, Glipizide, Glimepiride
   c. Meglitinide derivatives: Repaglinide, Nateglinide
   d. Alpha-glucosidase inhibitors: Acarbose
   e. Thiazolidinediones: Rosiglitazone, Pioglitazone
   f. Glucagon-like peptide 1 agonists: Exenatide, Liraglutide
   g. Dipeptidyl peptidase IV inhibitors: Sitagliptin, Linagliptin, Saxagliptin
   h. Selective sodium-glucose transporter 2 inhibitors: Dapagliflozin, Canagliflozin
   i. Insulin

B] Gynaecomastia

Points to remember

1. Causes:
   a. Physiological
   b. Klinefelter syndrome
   c. Kallmann syndrome
   d. Chronic renal failure
   e. Hyperthyroidism
   f. Pituitary tumours
   g. Medications:

   Cimetidine, Ketoconazole, Calcium channel blockers, anabolic steroids, 5 alpha-reductase inhibitors

Brief Clinical Consultations:
Ophthalmology

Case No 1: Diabetic Retinopathy

Points to remember

1. Non-proliferative retinopathy: Haemorrhages, microaneurysms and hard exudates
2. Proliferative retinopathy: All of above along with neovascularisation, tractional retinal detachment and macular oedema
3. Pharmacologic therapy: Triamcinolone, Bevacizumab
4. Other treatment modalities: Laser photocoagulation, vitrectomy, cryotherapy
5. Ensure adequate blood sugar control

Case No 2: Hypertensive Retinopathy

Points to remember

1. Keith-Wagener-Barker classification:
    a. Grade I: Slight narrowing, sclerosis and tortuosity of the retinal arterioles
    b. Grade II: Definite narrowing, constriction, sclerosis and AV nicking
    c. Grade III: Retinopathy - cotton wool patches, haemorrhages and arteriosclerosis
    d. Grade IV: Papilledema
2. Ensure adequate investigations for primary and secondary causes of
    hypertension
3. Ensure adequate management of hypertension

Case No 3: Retinitis Pigmentosa

Points to remember

1. Mainly progressive loss of peripheral vision with night vision disturbances leading to central vision loss

2. Most common form of inherited retinal degeneration due to progressive loss of photoreceptor cells, eventually leading to blindness

3. Syndromes associated with retinitis pigmentosa:

    a. Kearns-Sayre syndrome – Retinitis pigmentosa with ophthalmoplegia, dysphagia, ataxia and cardiac conduction defects

    b. Usher syndrome, Waardenburg syndrome, Refsum disease and Alport Syndrome - Retinitis pigmentosa with deafness

    c. Abetalipoproteinemia - Retinitis pigmentosa with intellectual impairment, peripheral neuropathy, ataxia and steatorrhea

    d. Bardet-Biedl syndrome - Retinitis pigmentosa with truncal obesity, polydactyly, renal dysfunction and short stature

Case No 4: Optic Atrophy

Points to remember

1. Optic nerve damage due to loss of retinal ganglion cell axons leading to the pale optic nerve on fundoscopy.

2. Causes:

    a. Hereditary: Behr and Leber hereditary optic atrophy

    b. Metabolic: Nutritional amblyopia, thyroid ophthalmopathy, diabetes, medications - ethambutol, sulphonamides, toxic amblyopia

    c. Demyelinating diseases - multiple sclerosis

    d. Post-inflammatory atrophy - optic neuritis

    e. Pressure or traction atrophy - glaucoma, papilledema

Case No 5: Myasthenia Gravis

Points to remember

1. Autoimmune neuromuscular disease due to circulating antibodies blocking the acetylcholine receptor at the post-synaptic neuromuscular junction
2. Hallmark of myasthenia is fatigability
3. Associated autoimmune conditions:

    Thyroid diseases, diabetes mellitus type 1, rheumatoid arthritis, and systemic lupus erythematosus
4. Blood tests: Anti-acetylcholine receptor antibody, anti-striated muscle antibody, anti-muscle-specific kinase antibody, and an autoimmune screen is essential
5. Decremental response to repetitive nerve stimulation is characteristic
6. Anticholinesterase or Edrophonium test is infrequently performed
7. Ice pack test for assessing improvement in ptosis and diplopia in ocular myasthenia gravis
8. Pharmacologic therapy:

    Anticholinesterase medication and immunosuppressive agents, such as corticosteroids, Azathioprine, Cyclosporine, plasmapheresis, and intravenous immune globulin
9. Thymectomy is also an option

Case No 6: Ocular palsy

Points to remember

1. III nerve palsy characteristically leaves the eye in a down and out position
2. Causes:
   a. Congenital causes
   b. Vascular causes: Diabetes, atherosclerosis, posterior communicating artery aneurysm
   c. Demyelinating diseases
   d. Autoimmune disease
   e. Inflammation
   f. Infection
   g. Cavernous sinus thrombosis
   h. Trauma

Case No 7: Old Choroiditis

Points to remember

1. Common aetiologies: Cytomegalovirus, toxoplasmosis
2. Other causes: Immunocompromised states - Acquired immune deficiency syndrome, other infections - Lyme disease, candida, yersinia and tuberculosis
3. Treatment involves treating the primary pathology

Case No 8: Retinal Artery/ Vein Occlusion

Points to remember

1. Painless loss of vision is a common presenting complaint for retinal artery occlusion
2. A complete visual field defect goes in favour of the central retinal artery occlusion and a sectional defect indicate a branch retinal artery occlusion
3. Causes for retinal artery occlusion:
    a. Embolic causes
    b. Inflammatory causes
    c. Thrombophilia
    d. Carotid artery dissection
4. Causes for retinal vein occlusion:
    a. Hypertension, diabetes
    b. Atherosclerosis
    c. Hypercholesterolaemia, hyperhomocystinemia
    d. Waldenstroms macroglobulinemia

Case No 9: Visual Field Defect

Aetiology

1. Cerebrovascular accident
2. Tumours:
   a. Craniopharyngioma
   b. Pituitary tumour
   c. Glioma
   d. Meningioma
3. Hydrocephalus
4. Drugs: e.g. Vigabatrin
5. Ocular causes: Glaucoma, macular degeneration, retinitis pigmentosa, optic neuritis, Leber's optic atrophy, ischaemic optic neuropathy
6. Demyelination
7. Vascular causes:
8. Others: Migraine, vasculitis, nutritional deficiencies, toxins

Management

Investigations

Blood Tests

1. Full blood count
2. Renal function
3. Liver function

4. ESR
5. CRP
6. Autoimmune screen, serum caeruloplasmin
7. Vitamin B12/ folic acid levels
8. Vasculitic screen
9. Thyroid function tests
10. Fasting blood glucose and HbA1C
11. Lipids
12. Serum protein electrophoresis, immunoglobulins
13. Homocysteine level
14. Cardiac biomarkers
15. Drug levels
16. Blood cultures

Imaging Studies

1. CT + CTA brain
2. MRI + MRA + MRV brain
3. Carotid dopplers
4. Echocardiogram
5. Chest X-ray
6. ECG
7. Perimetry

Other Investigations

1. Lumbar puncture

Treatment

General Measures

1. Patient education and advice
2. Promoting a healthy lifestyle - diet/ exercise/ stop smoking
3. Look at reversible causes - Cutting down on alcohol intake, advice against recreational drug use

Specific Measures

1. Refer to a neurologist/ stroke physician
2. Referral to an ophthalmologist for ocular causes
3. Managing secondary risk factors - Hypertension/ diabetes/ hypercholesterolaemia
4. Multi-disciplinary team involvement - Physiotherapy, occupational therapy, speech and language therapy, social services
5. Treatment of any underlying cause

Case No 10: Other Cases

A] Cataracts

Points to remember

1. Types of cataracts:
    a. Congenital
    b. Nuclear
    c. Cortical
    d. Posterior subcapsular
2. Treatment options:
    a. Intracapsular cataract extraction
    b. Extracapsular cataract extraction
    c. Phacoemulsification
3. Remember to cover systemic diseases like diabetes and hypertension

B] Glaucoma

Points to remember

1. Types:
a. Open-angle glaucoma
b. Angle-closure glaucoma
2. Tonometric measurement of intraocular pressure of more than 21mmHg accounts for the diagnosis of glaucoma

3. Treatment:

a. Prostaglandin analogues: Latanoprost, Travoprost

b. Topical beta blockers: Timolol, Levobunolol

c. Alpha 2 adrenergic agonists: Brimonidine

d. Carbonic anhydrase inhibitors: Acetazolamide, Dorzolamide

e. Surgery:
Laser treatment, canaloplasty, trabeculectomy

C] Abnormal Pupils

Points to remember

1. Holmes-Adie pupil: Abnormally mydriatic pupil that does not constrict on exposure to light

2. Holmes-Adie syndrome: Holmes-Adie pupil with loss of deep tendon reflexes and abnormal sweating

3. Horner's syndrome: Ptosis, miosis, anhidrosis and enophthalmos
Causes may be classified according to the order of neuron involvement

   1. First-order neuron lesions:
   - Demyelinating disease
   - Pituitary tumour
   - Cerebrovascular accident
   - Basal meningitis
   - Syringomyelia

   2. Second-order neuron lesions:
   - Pancoast's tumour
   - Cervical rib
   - Central venous cannulation
   - Lymphadenopathy

3. Third-order neuron lesions:
- Internal carotid artery dissection
- Carotid cavernous fistula
- Migraine
- Herpes zoster

4 Argyll Robertson pupil: Preserved accommodation reflex with loss of light reflex
- Highly specific for neurosyphilis

5. III nerve palsy: Ptosis with a downward and outward deviation of the affected eye
- Causes: Infarction, infection, inflammation, haemorrhage, neoplasm, abscess

C] Age-Related Macular Degeneration

Points to remember

1. Types:
- Wet or exudative macular degeneration
- Dry or non-exudative macular degeneration
2. Dry macular degeneration characteristically shows drusen on fundoscopy, which accumulates between the choroid and retina, leading to retinal detachment
3. Wet macular degeneration causes vision loss due to choroidal neovascularisation ultimately leading to retinal detachment